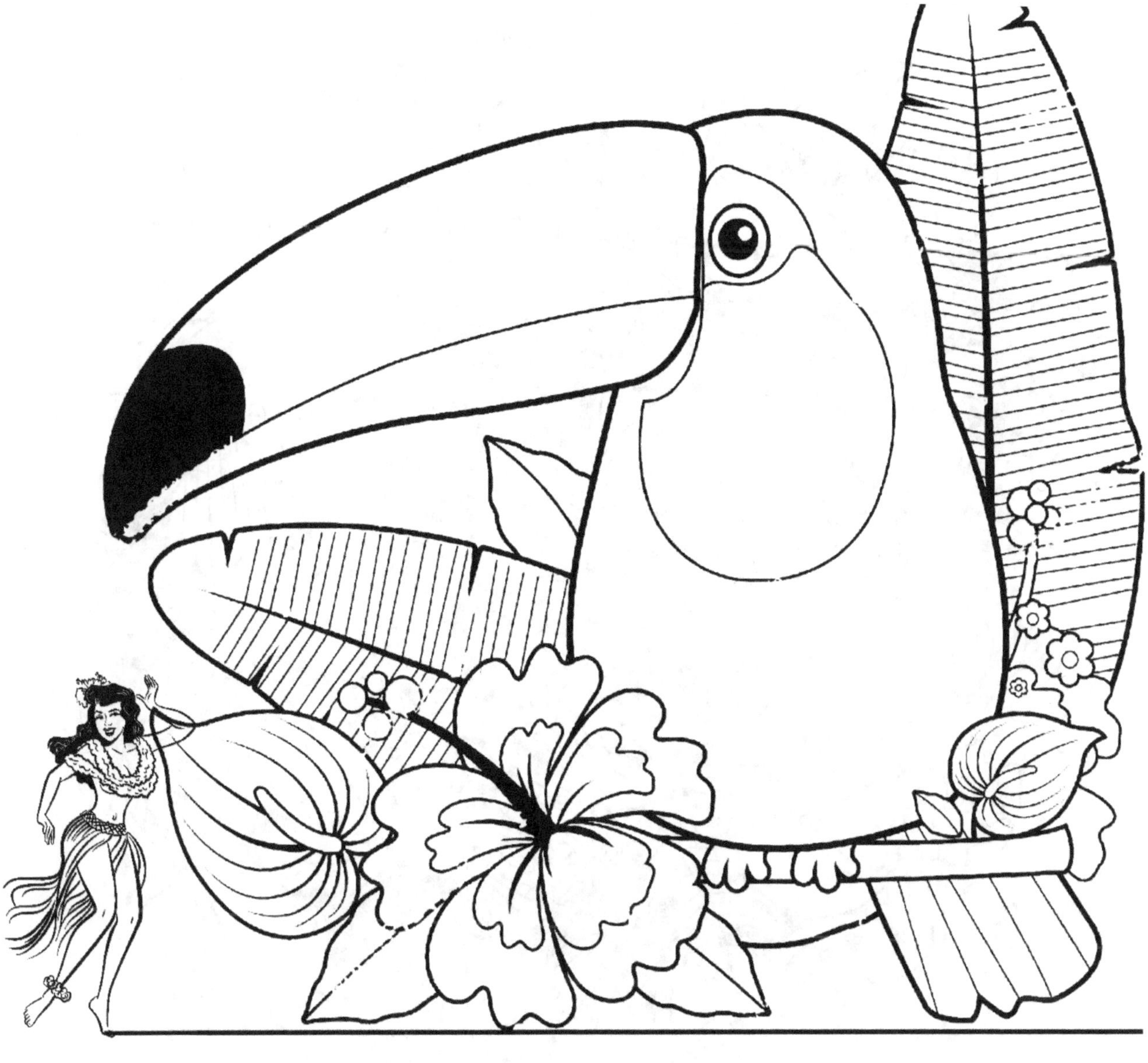

This Book Belongs To

....

....

....

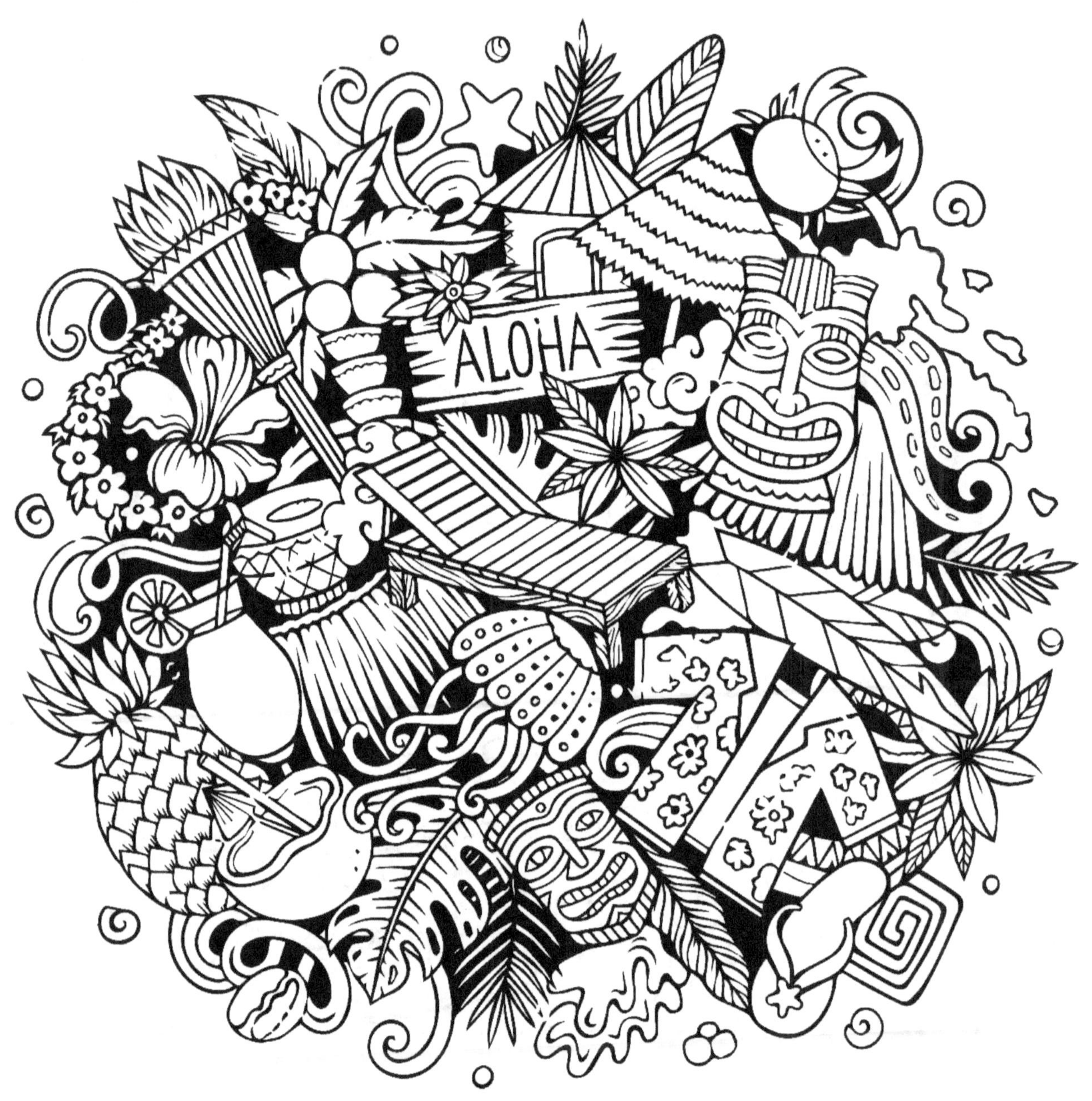

Coloring Page For Relax and Relief

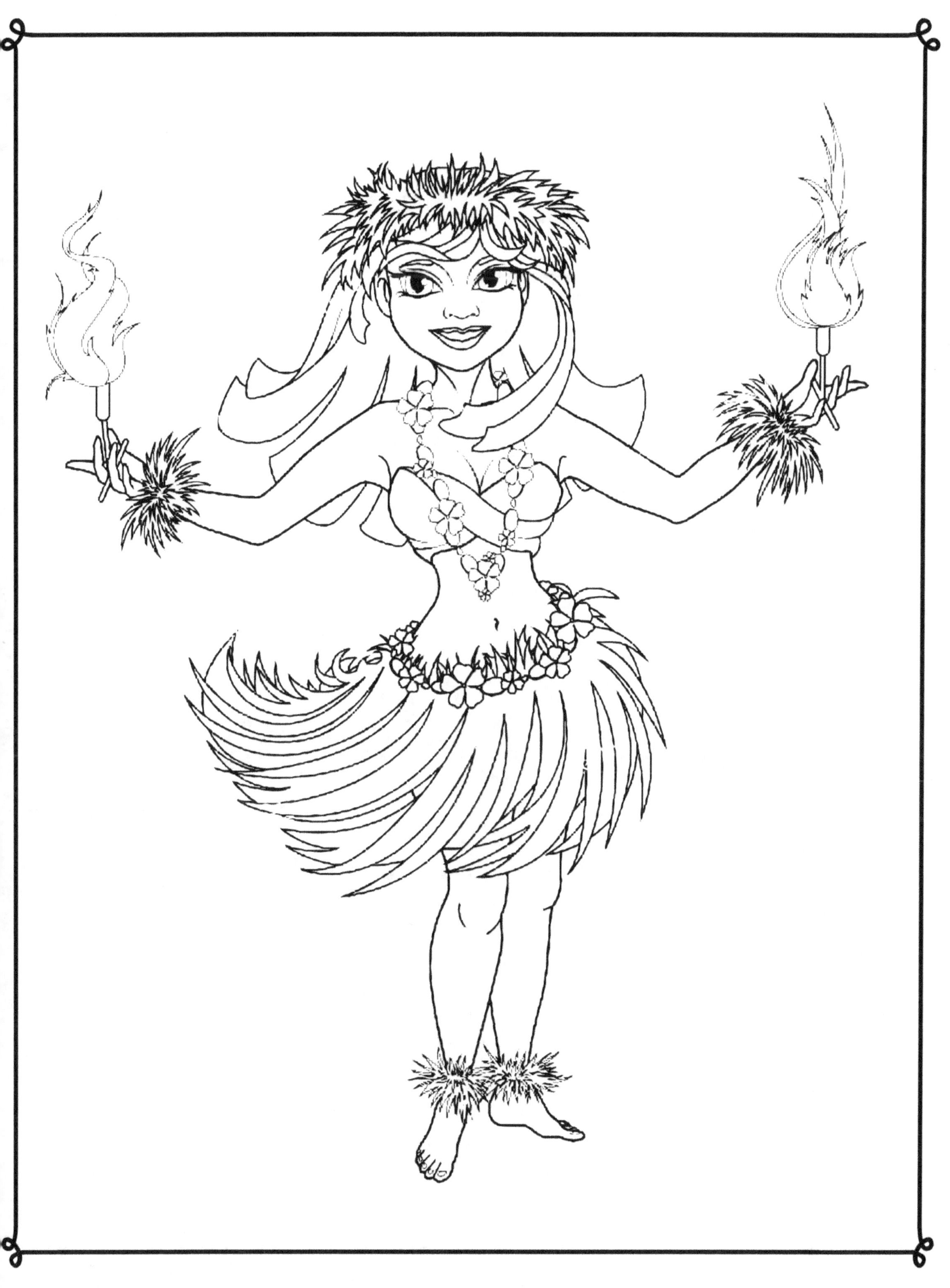

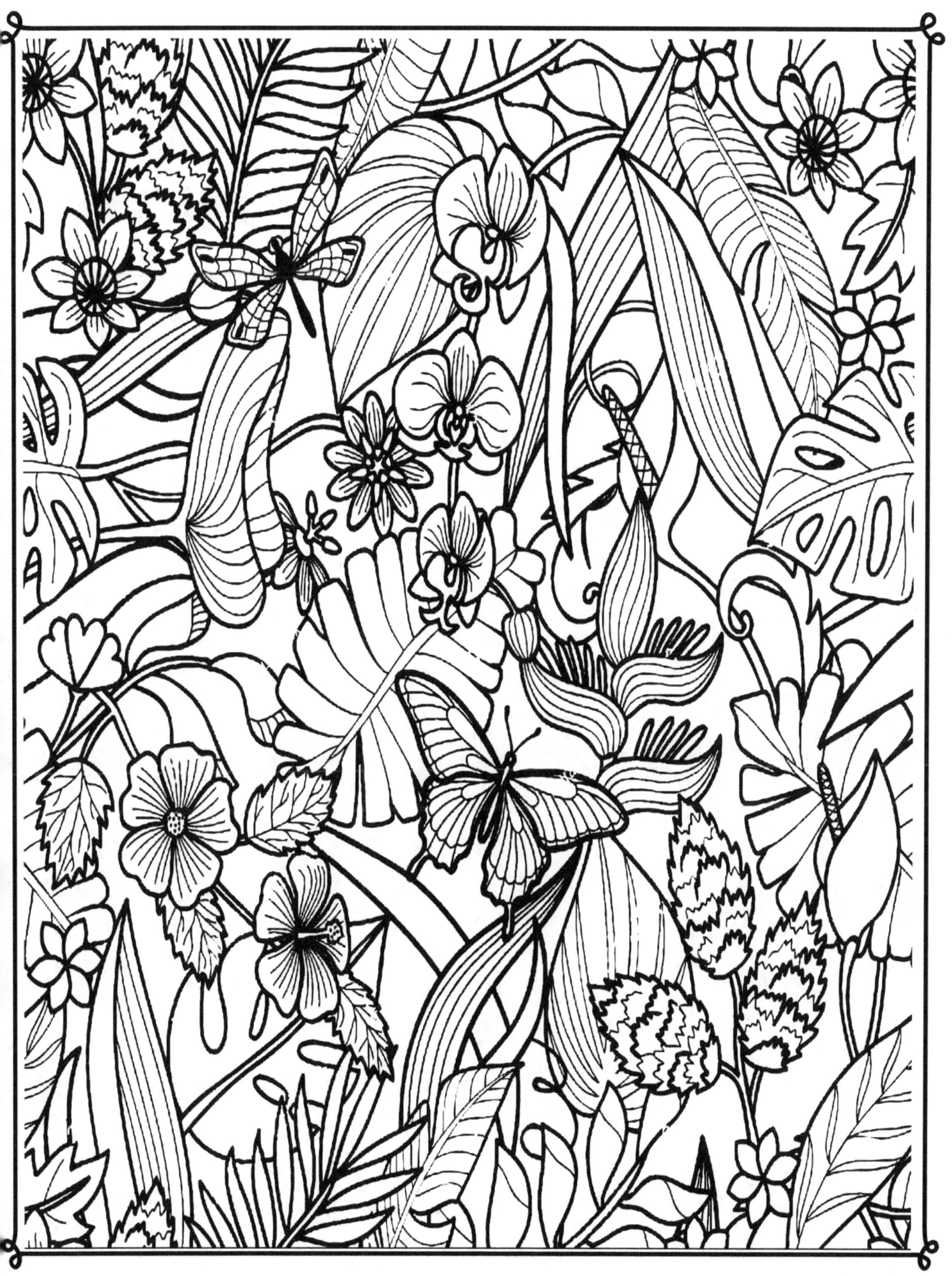

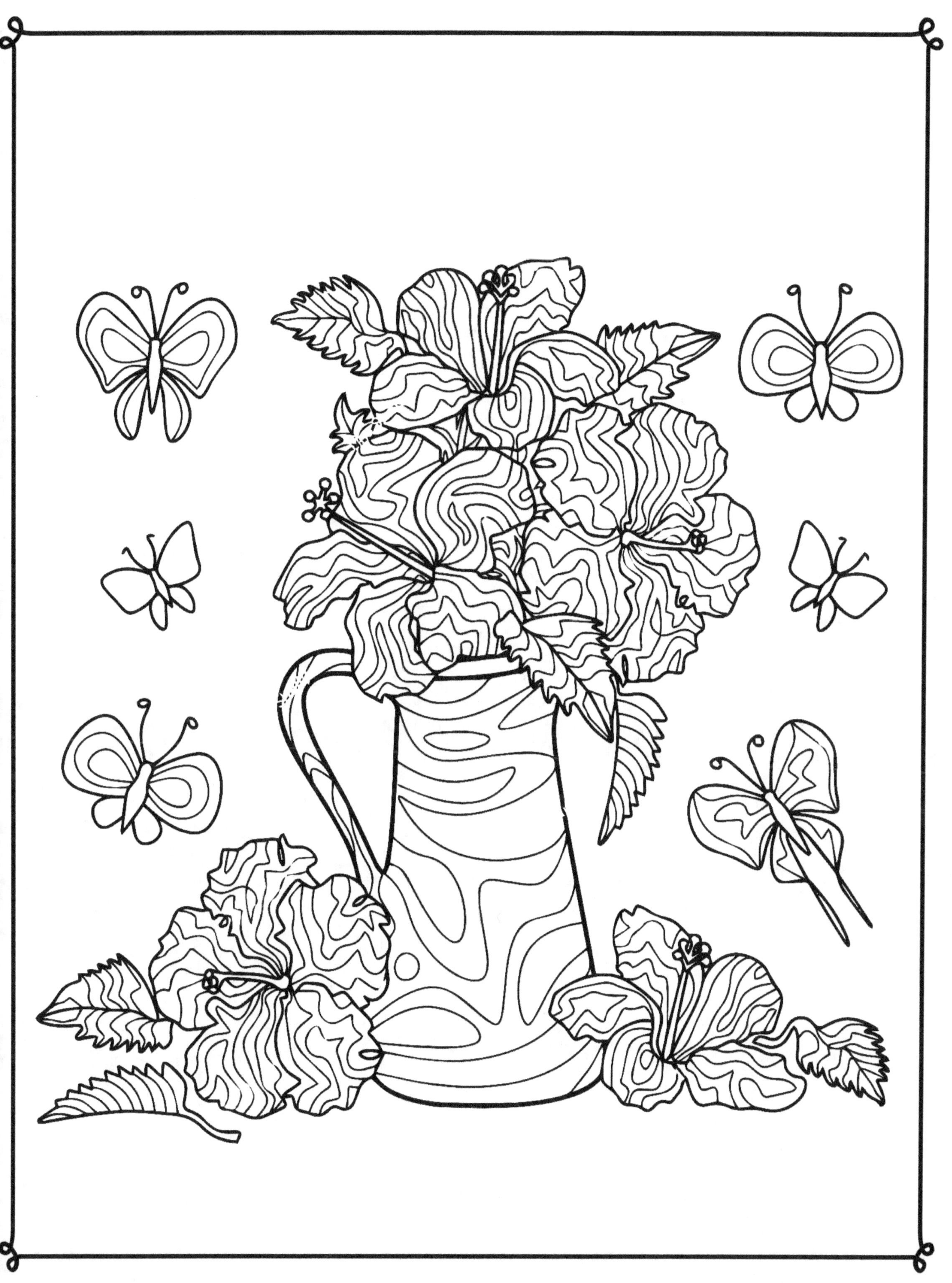

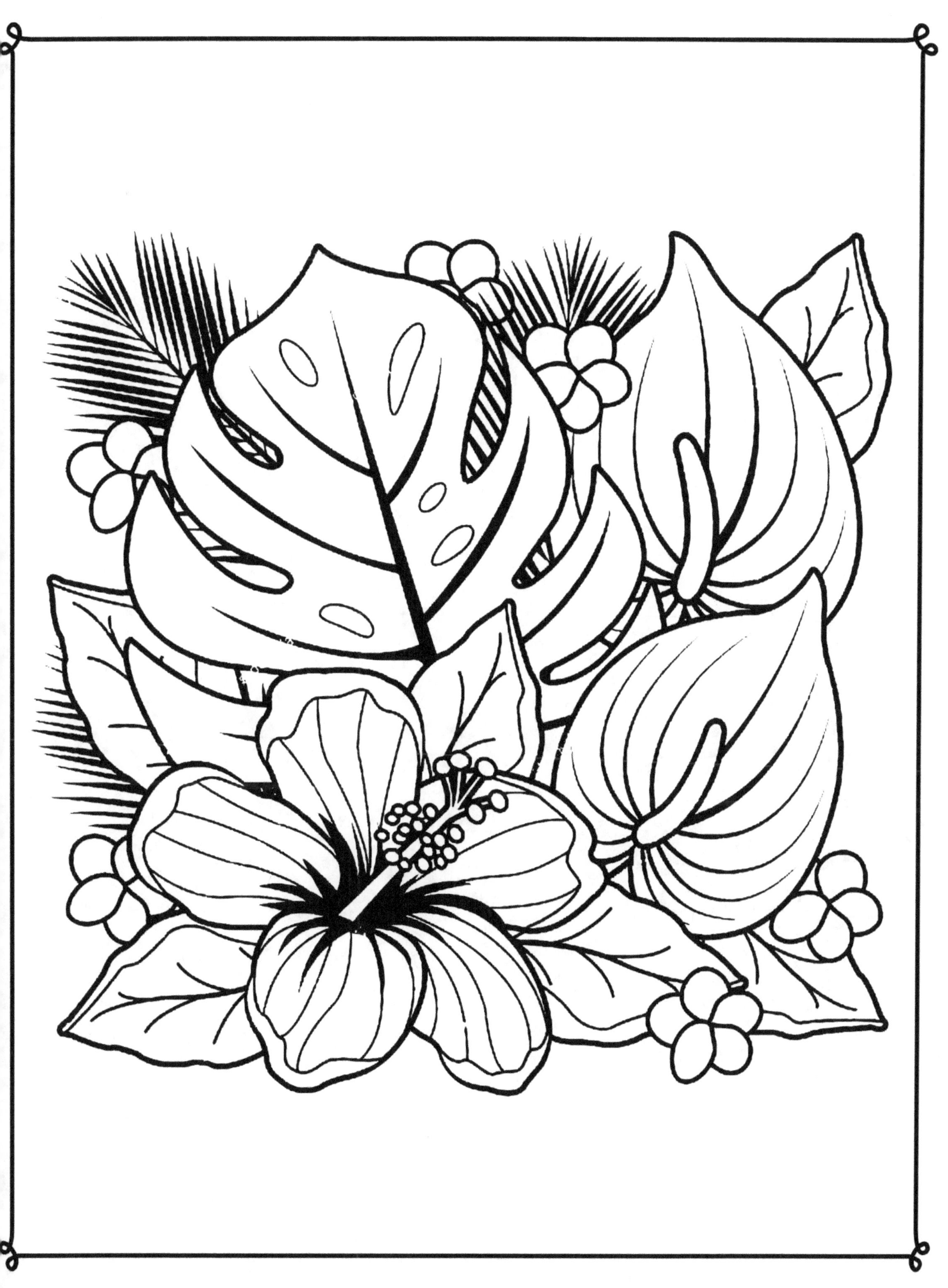

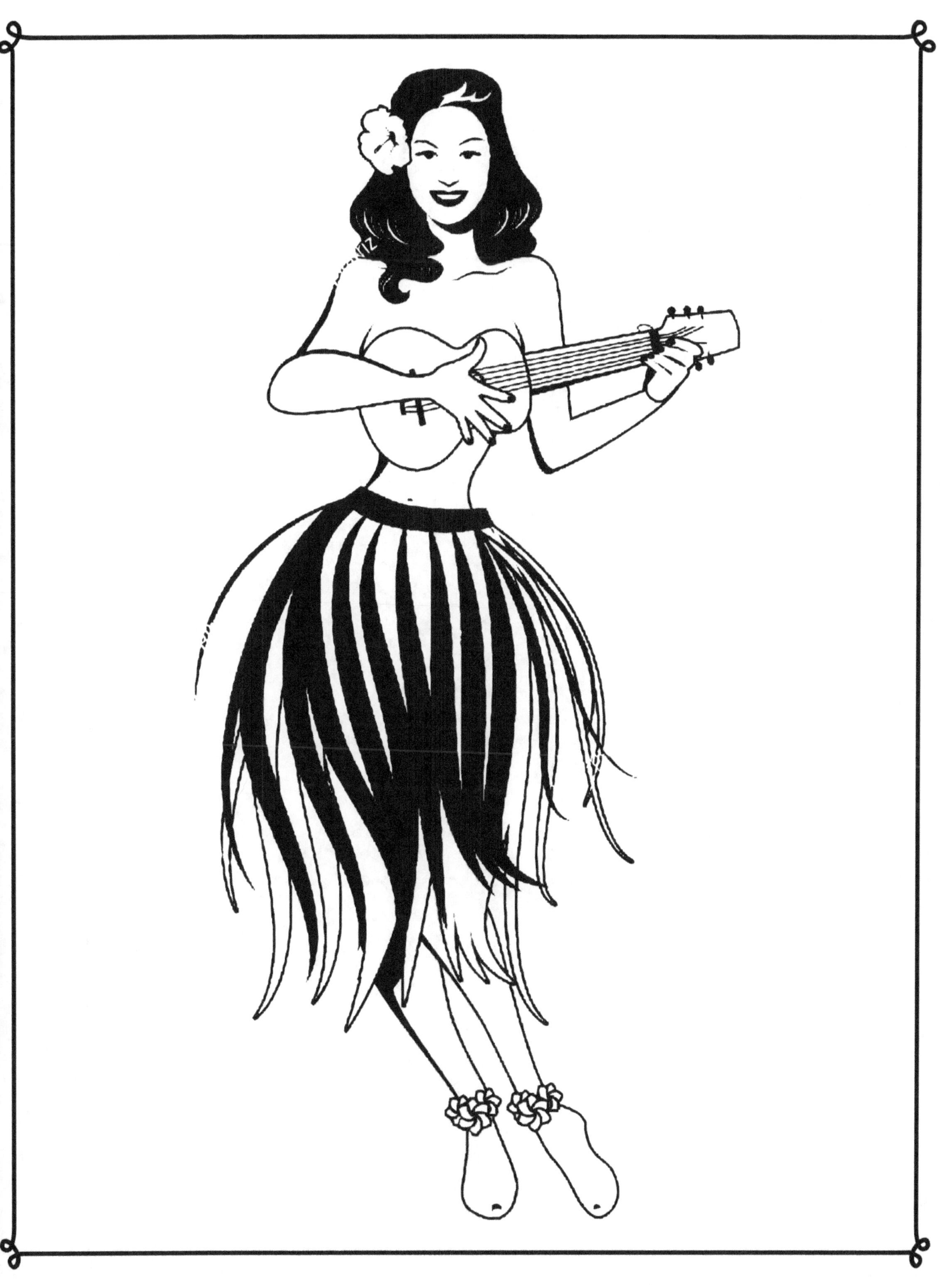

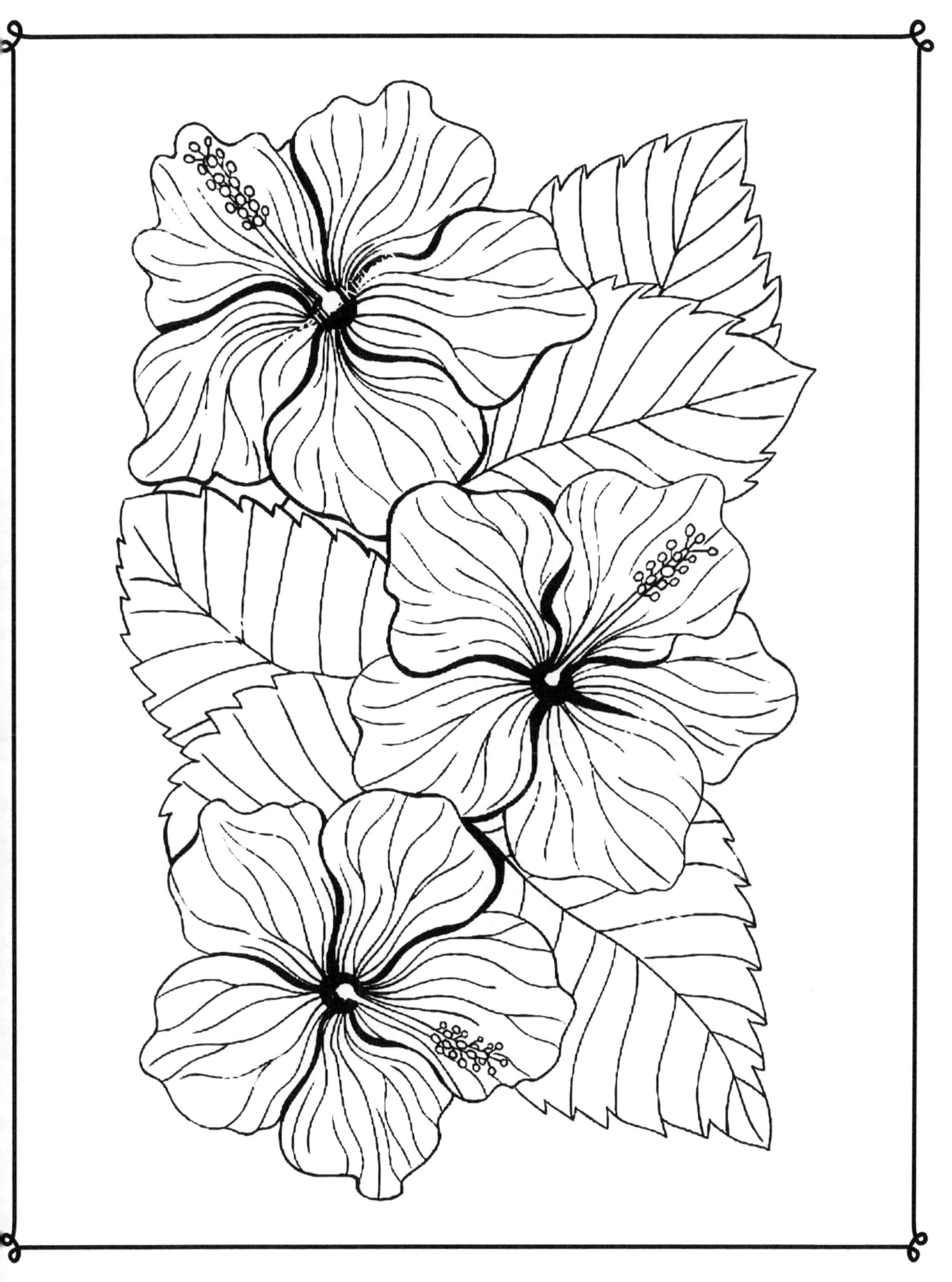

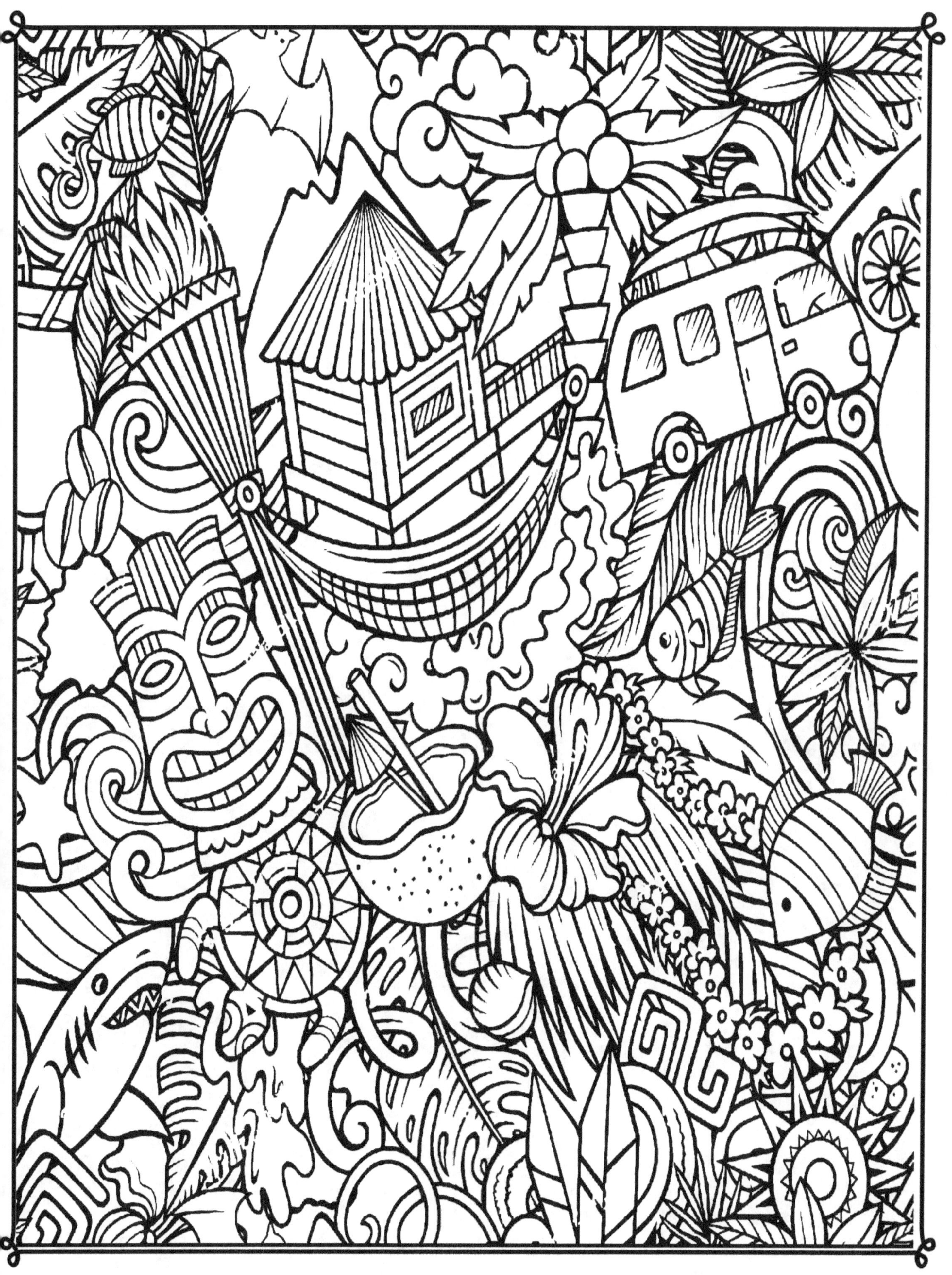

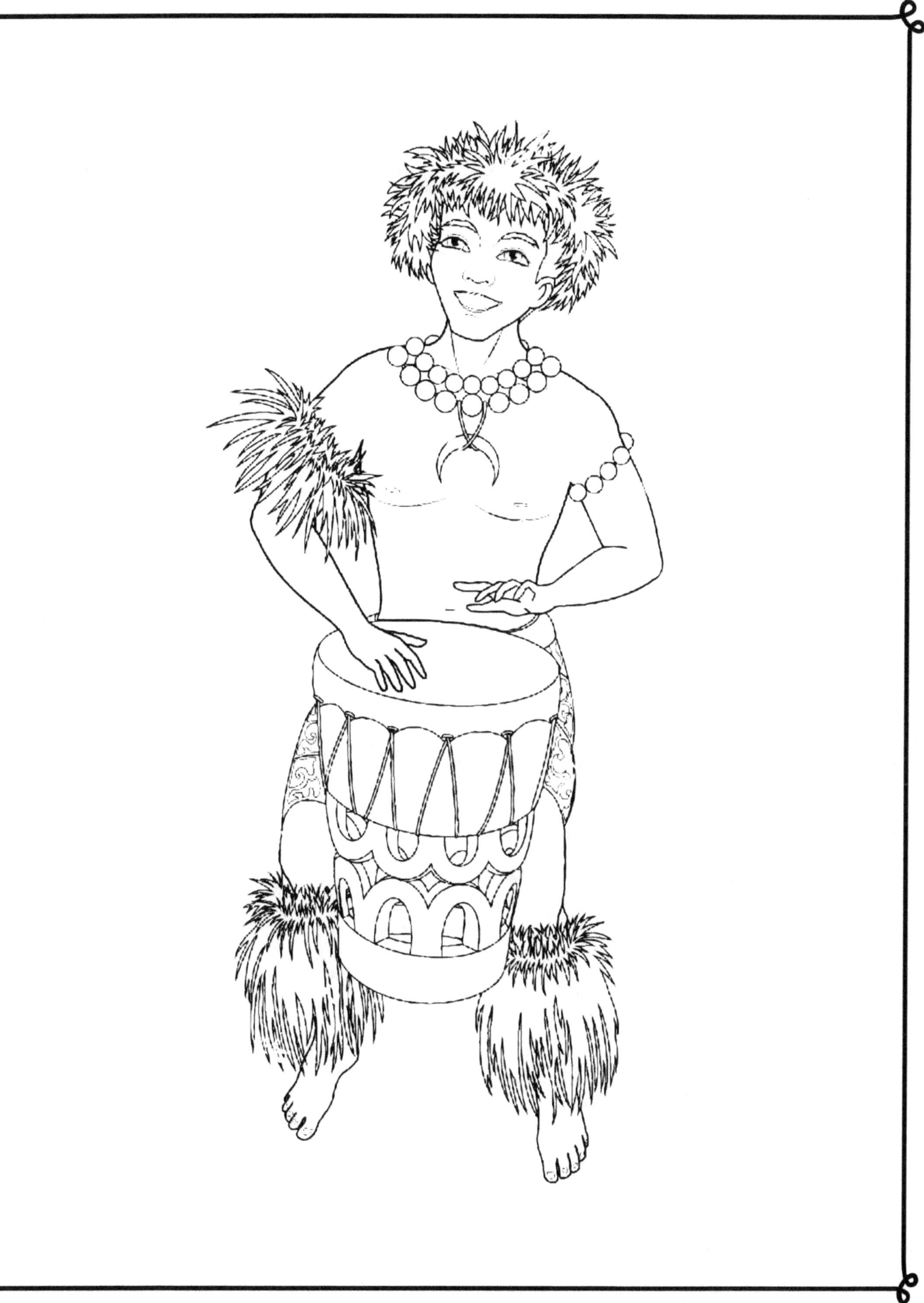

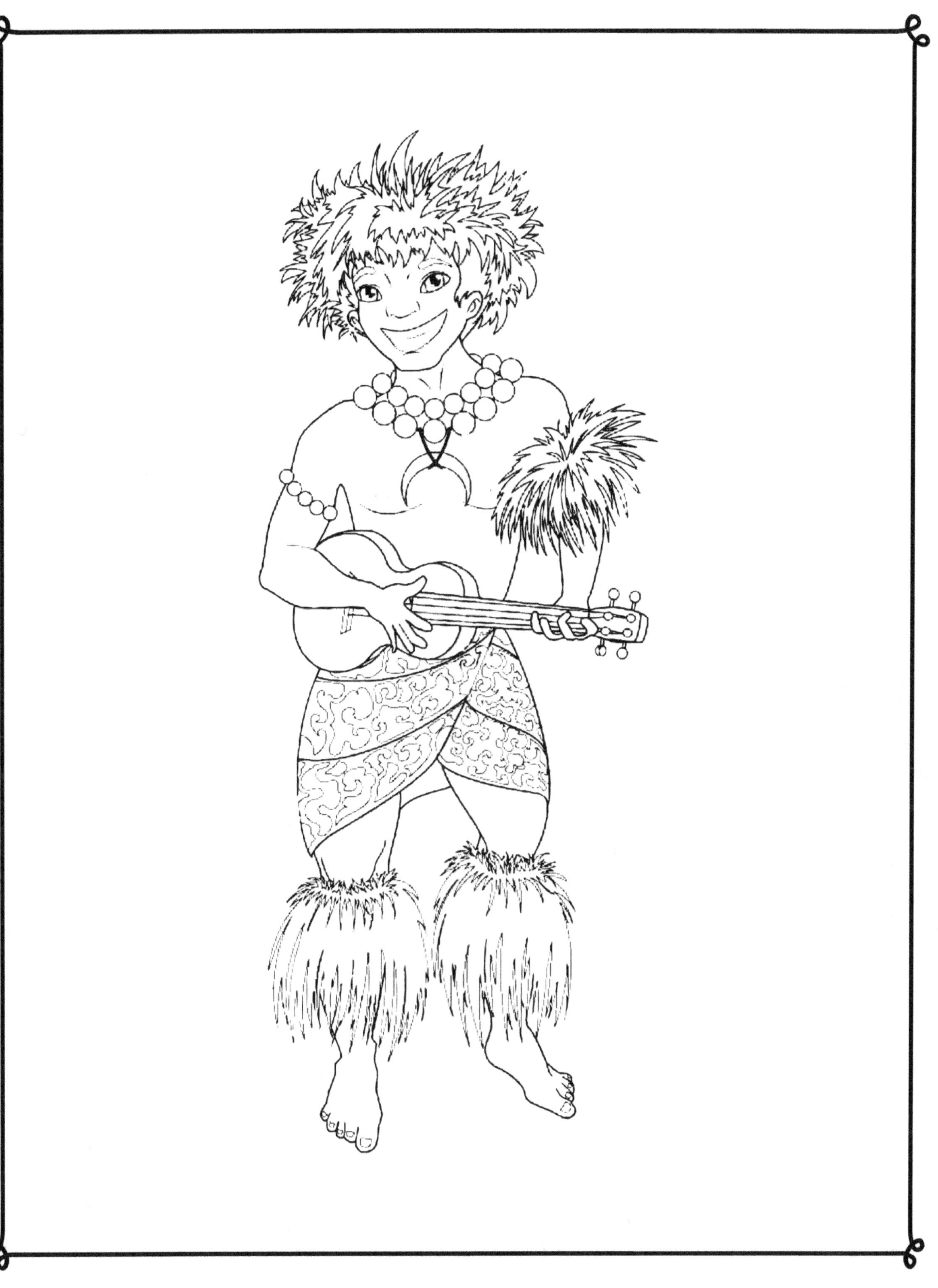

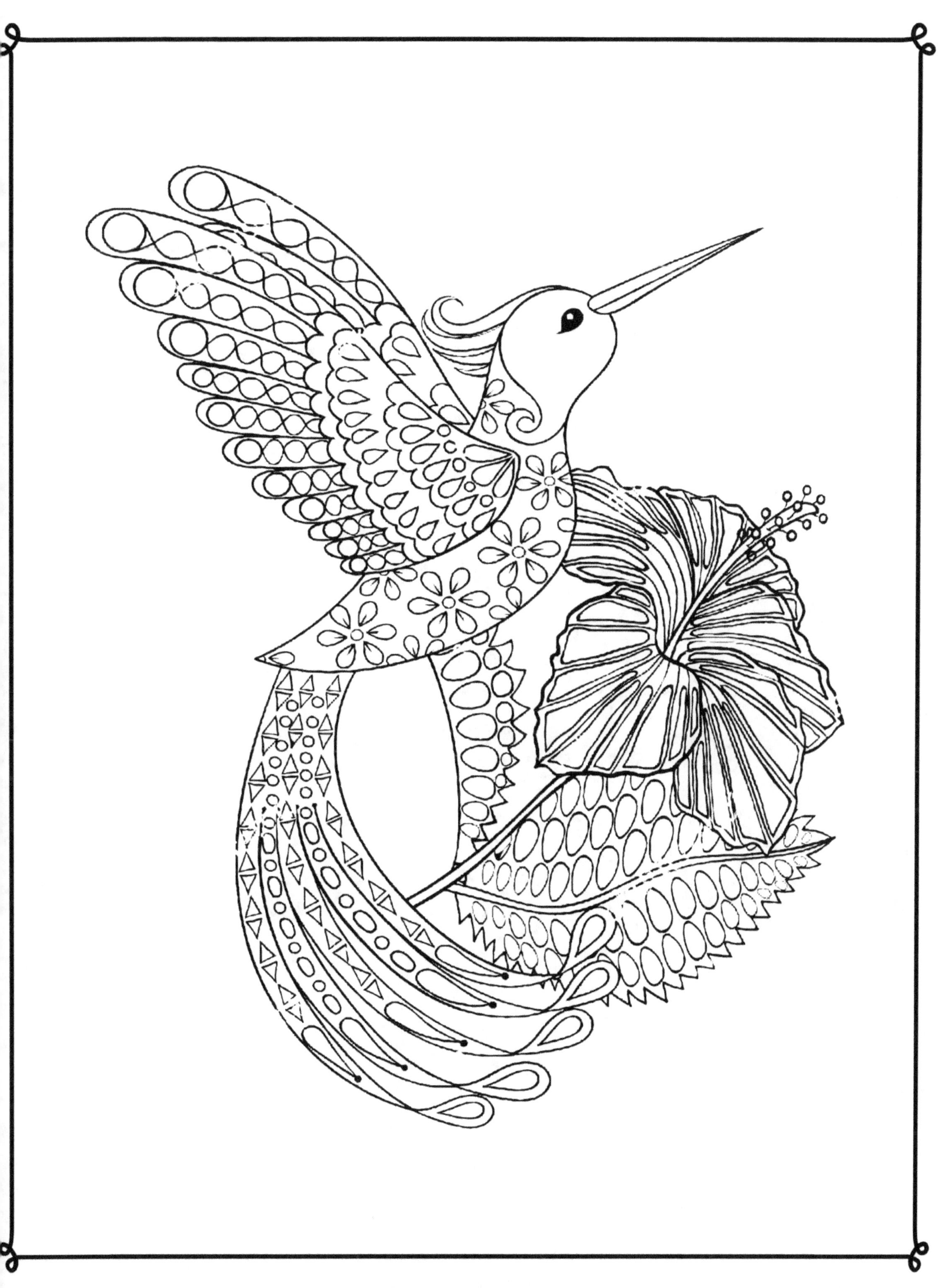

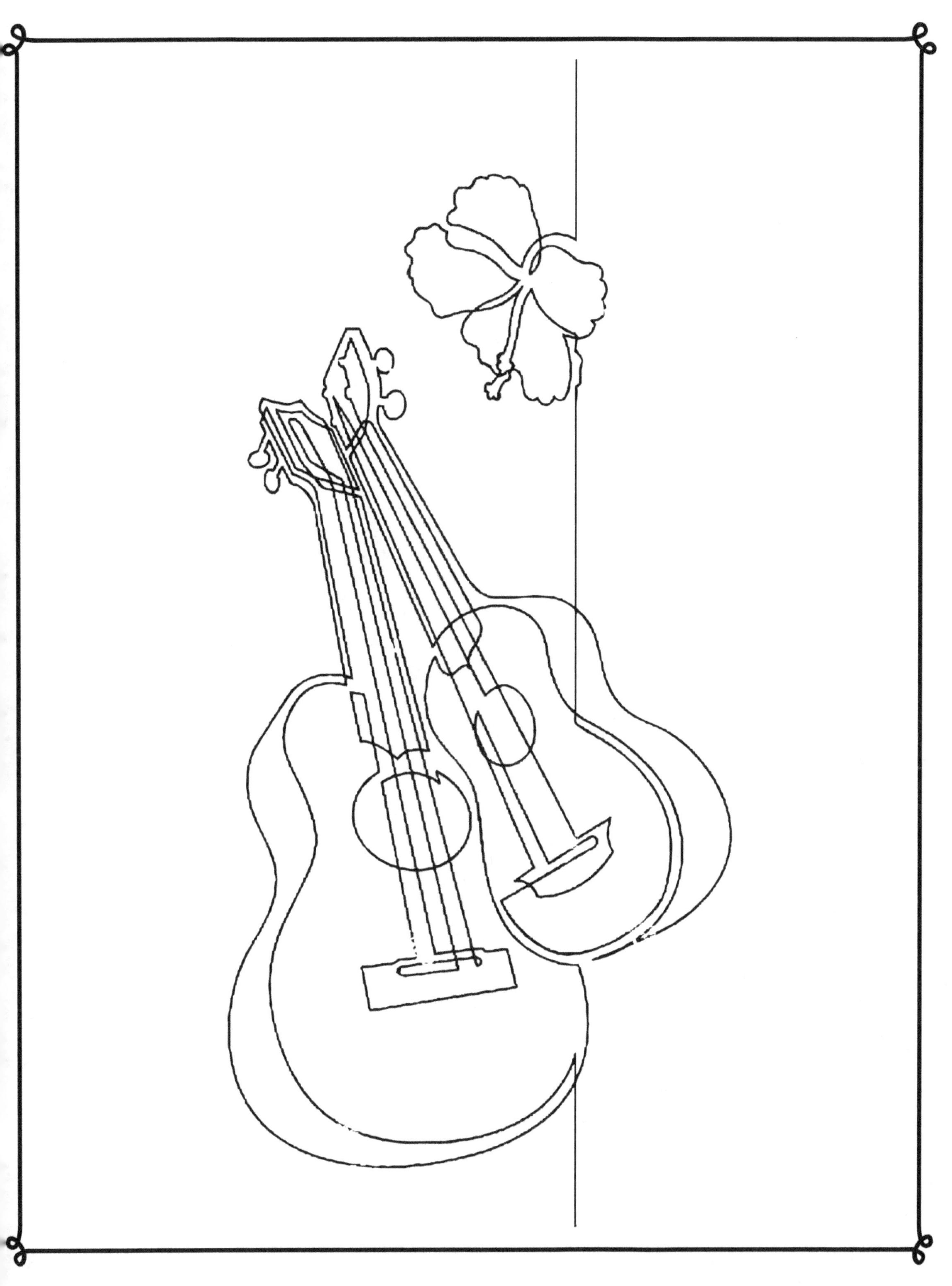

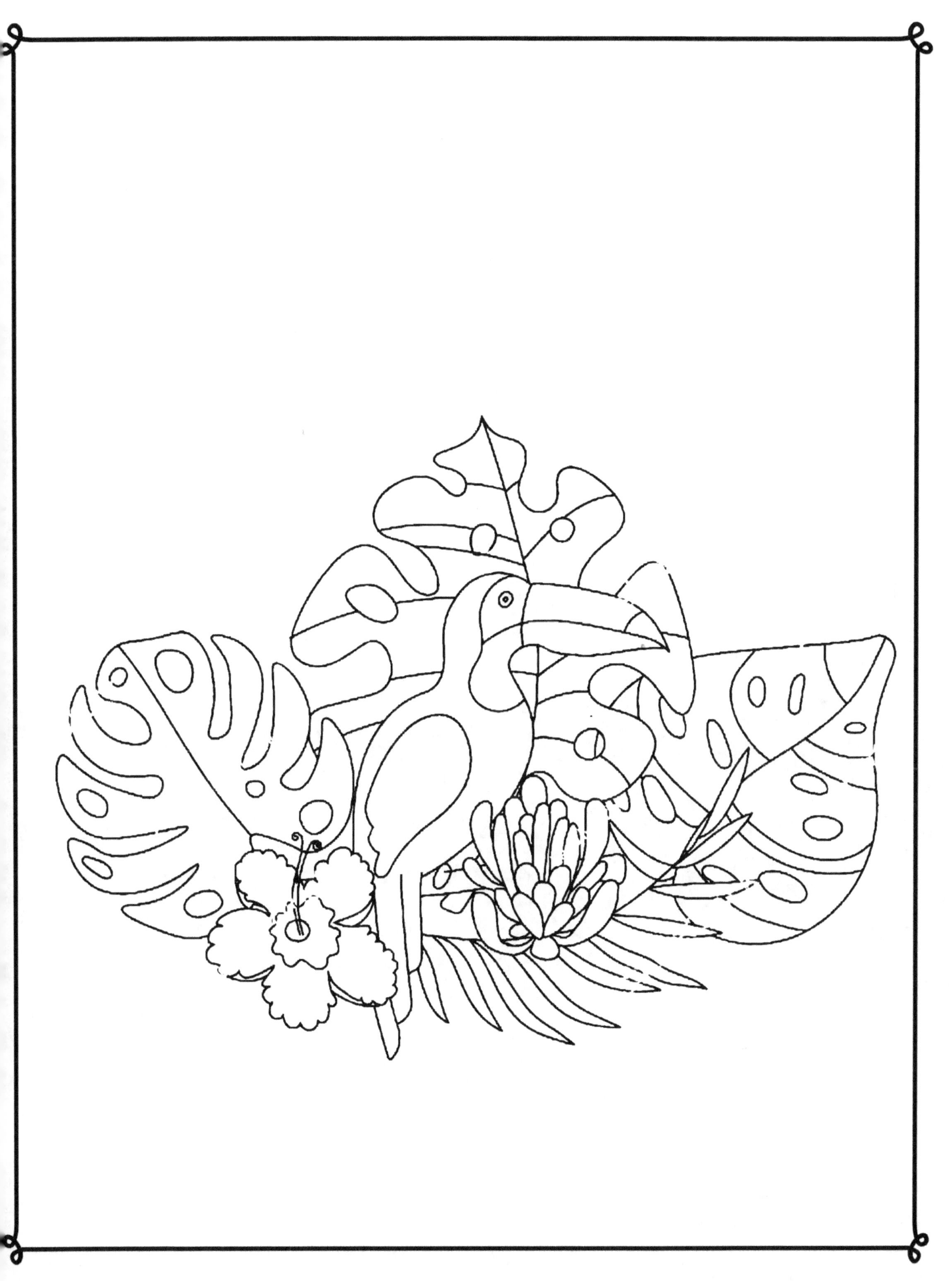

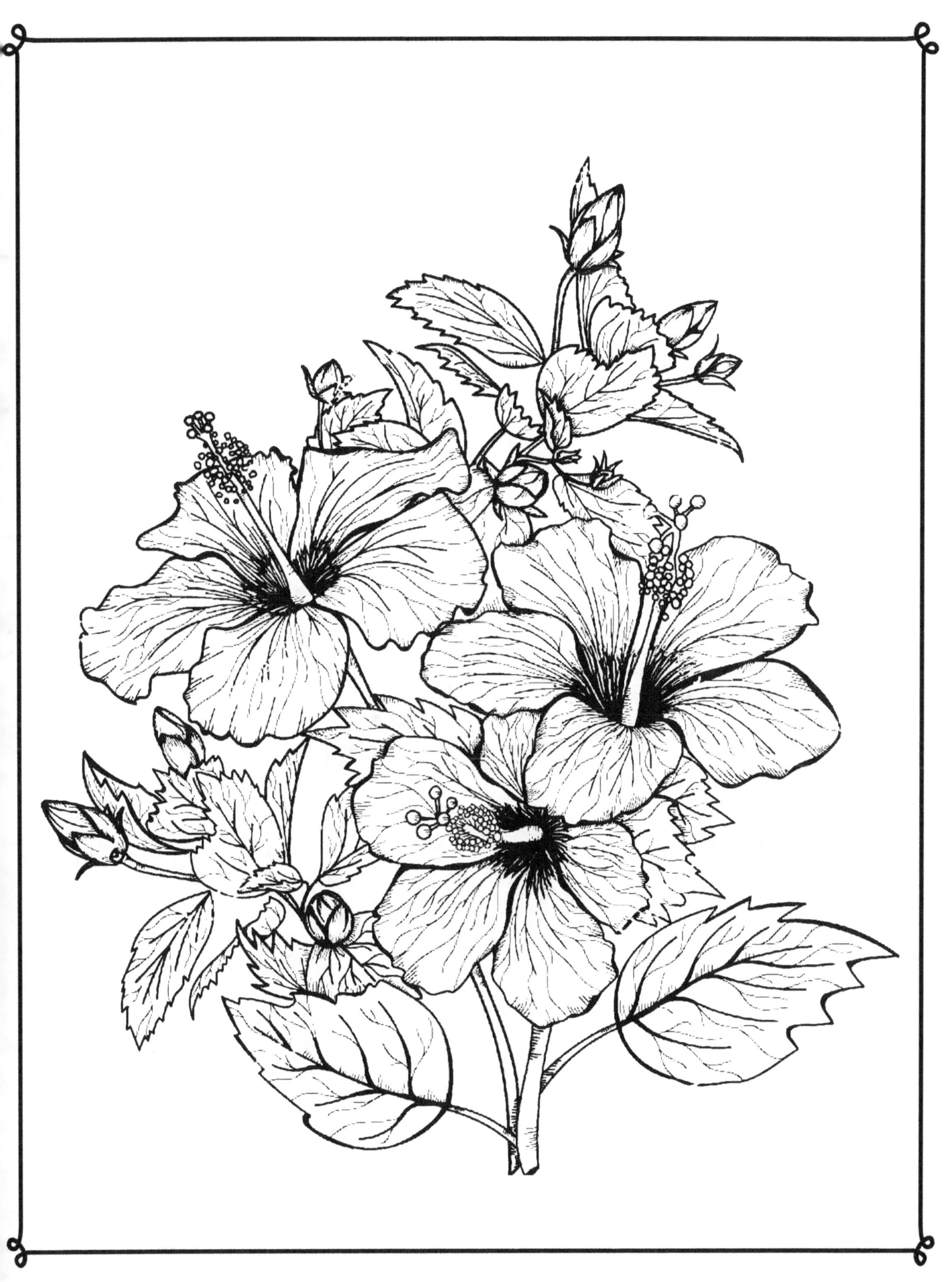

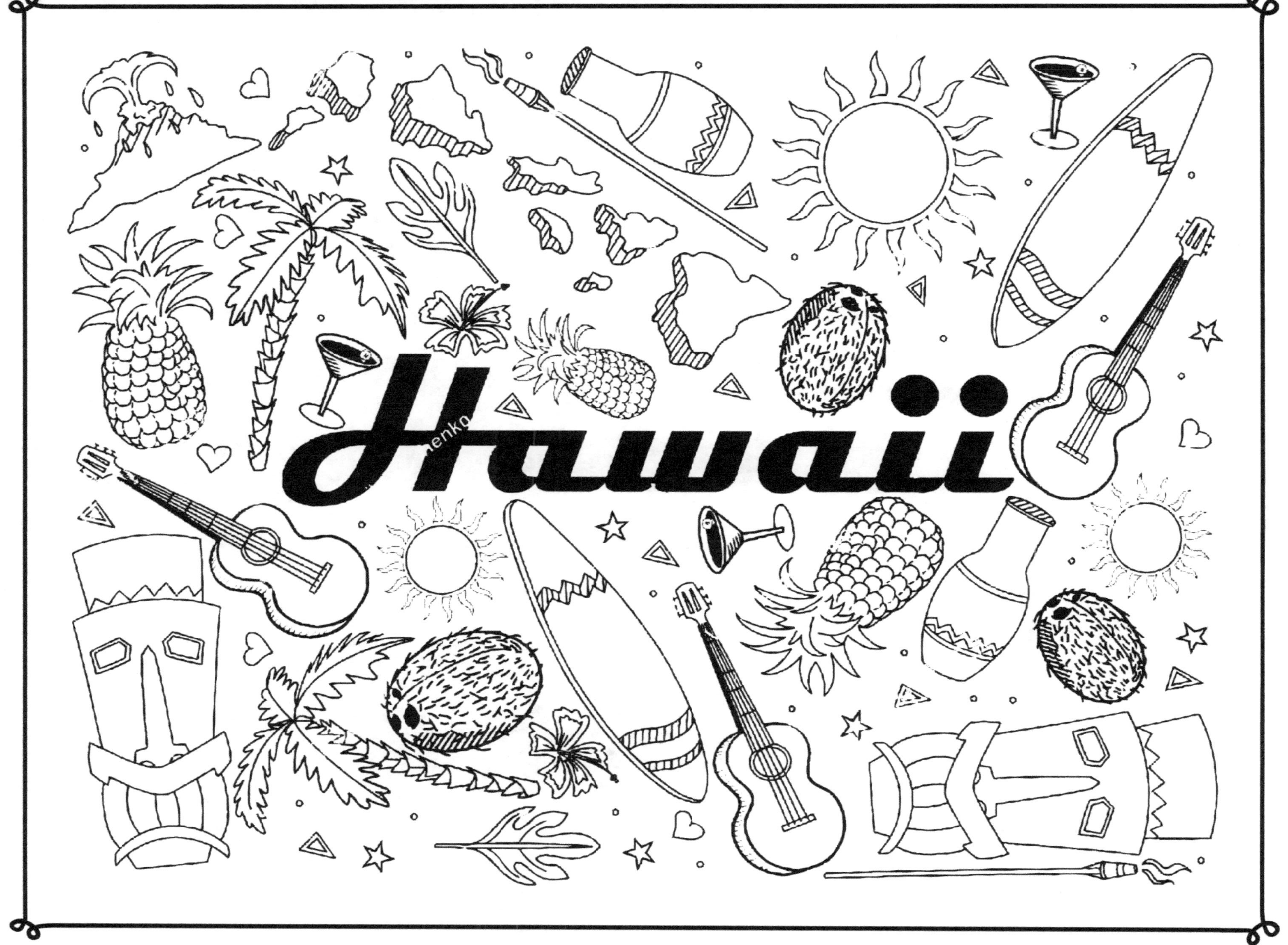

Hawaii

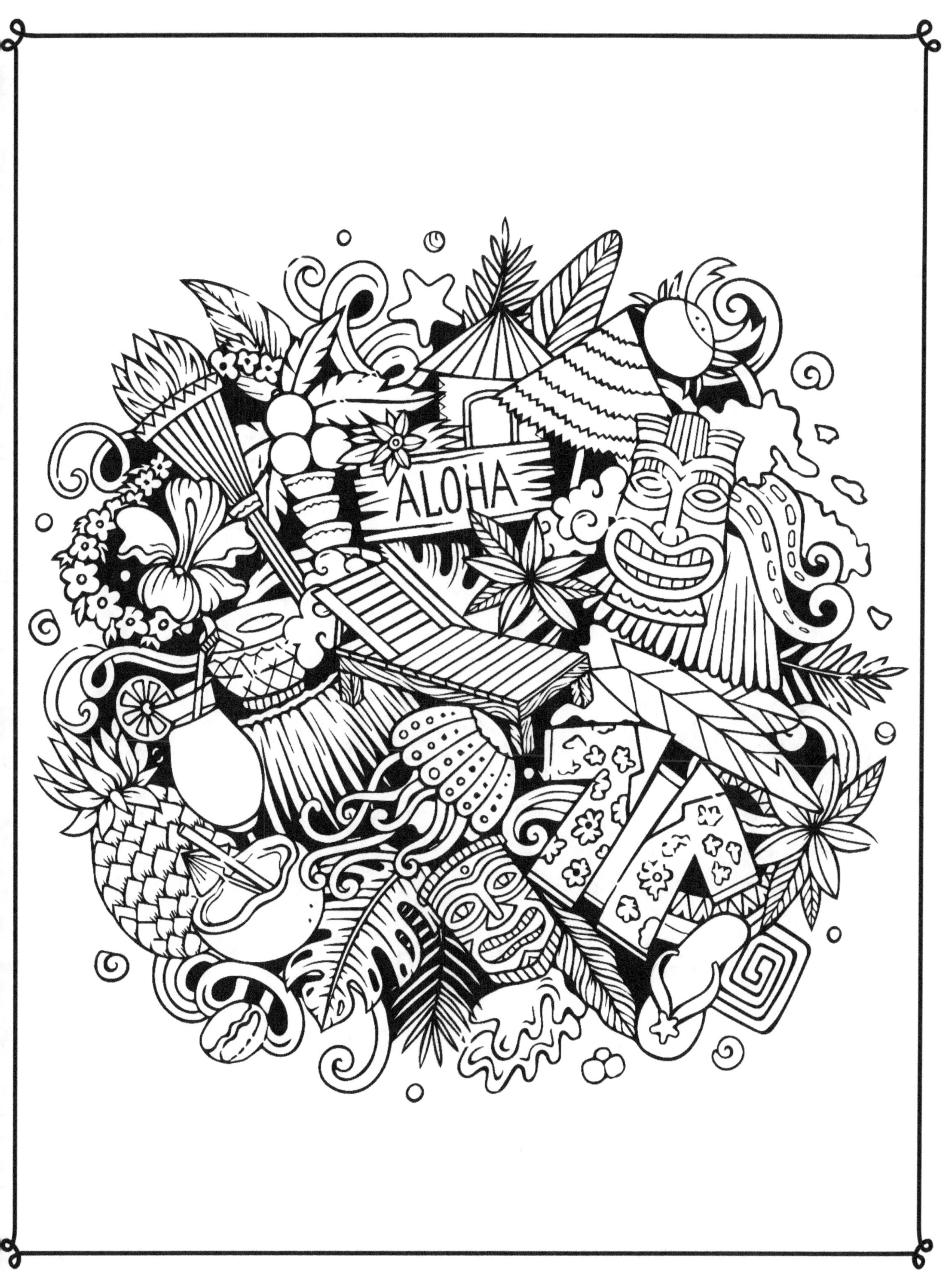

ALOHA

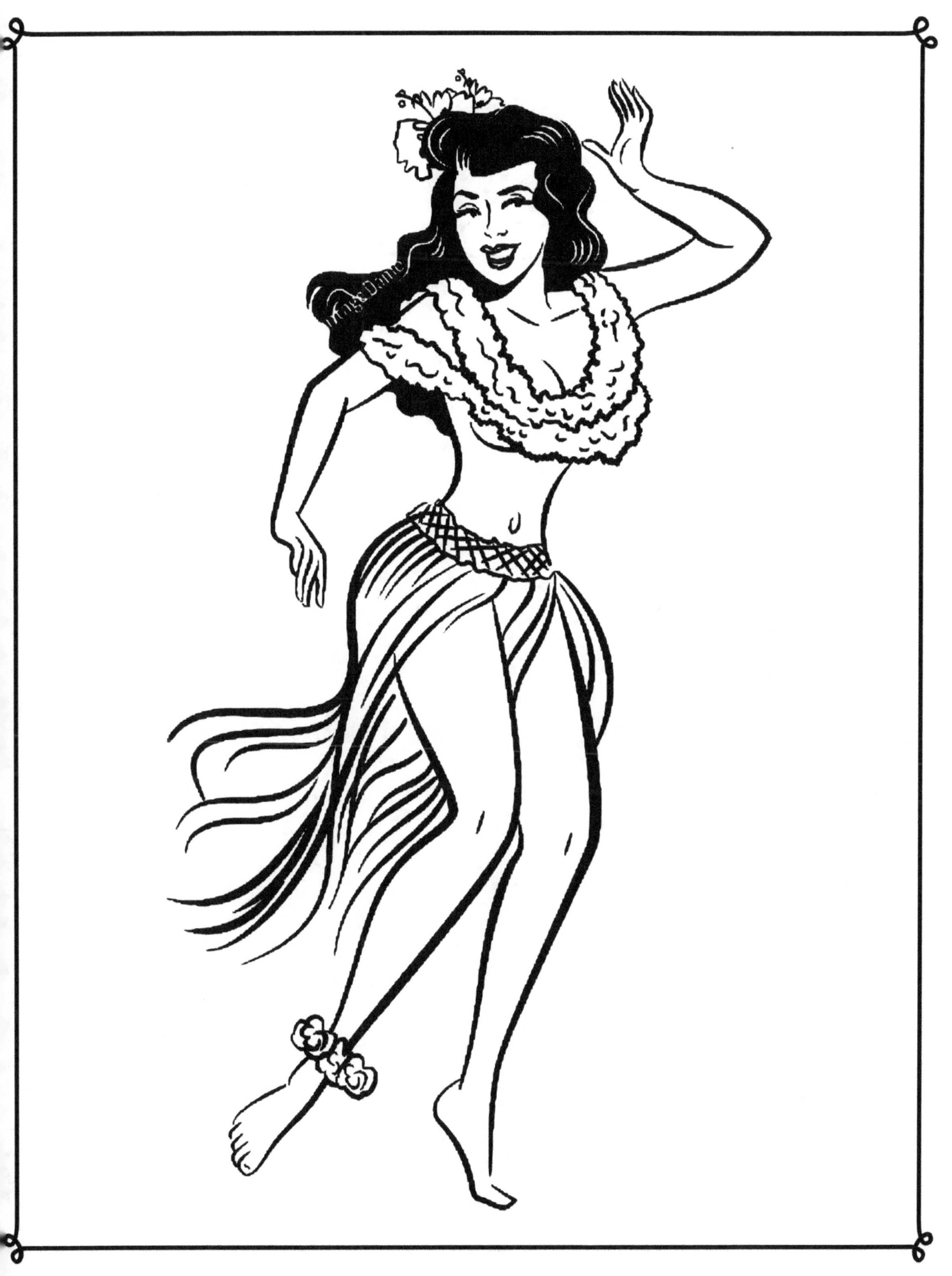

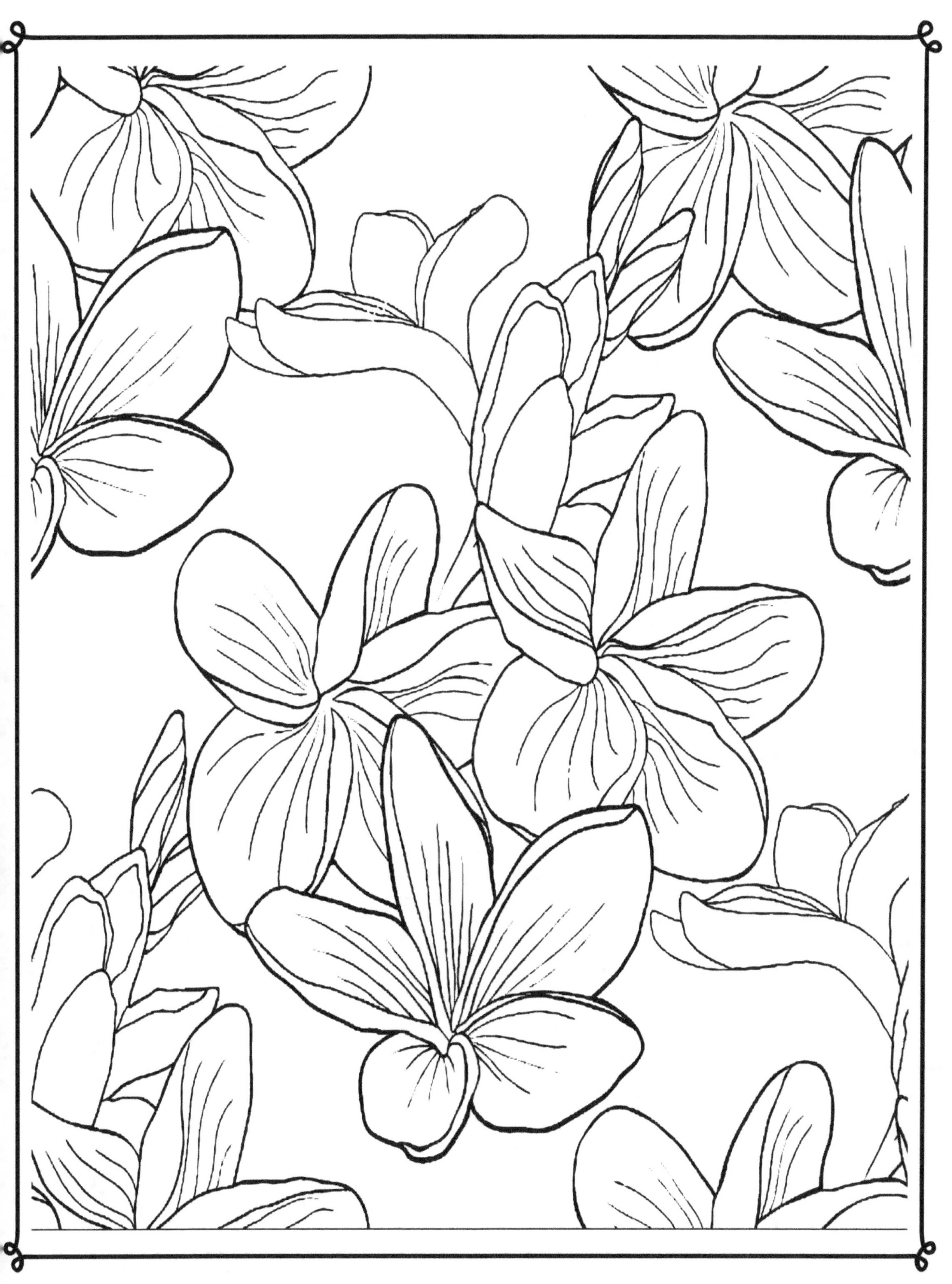

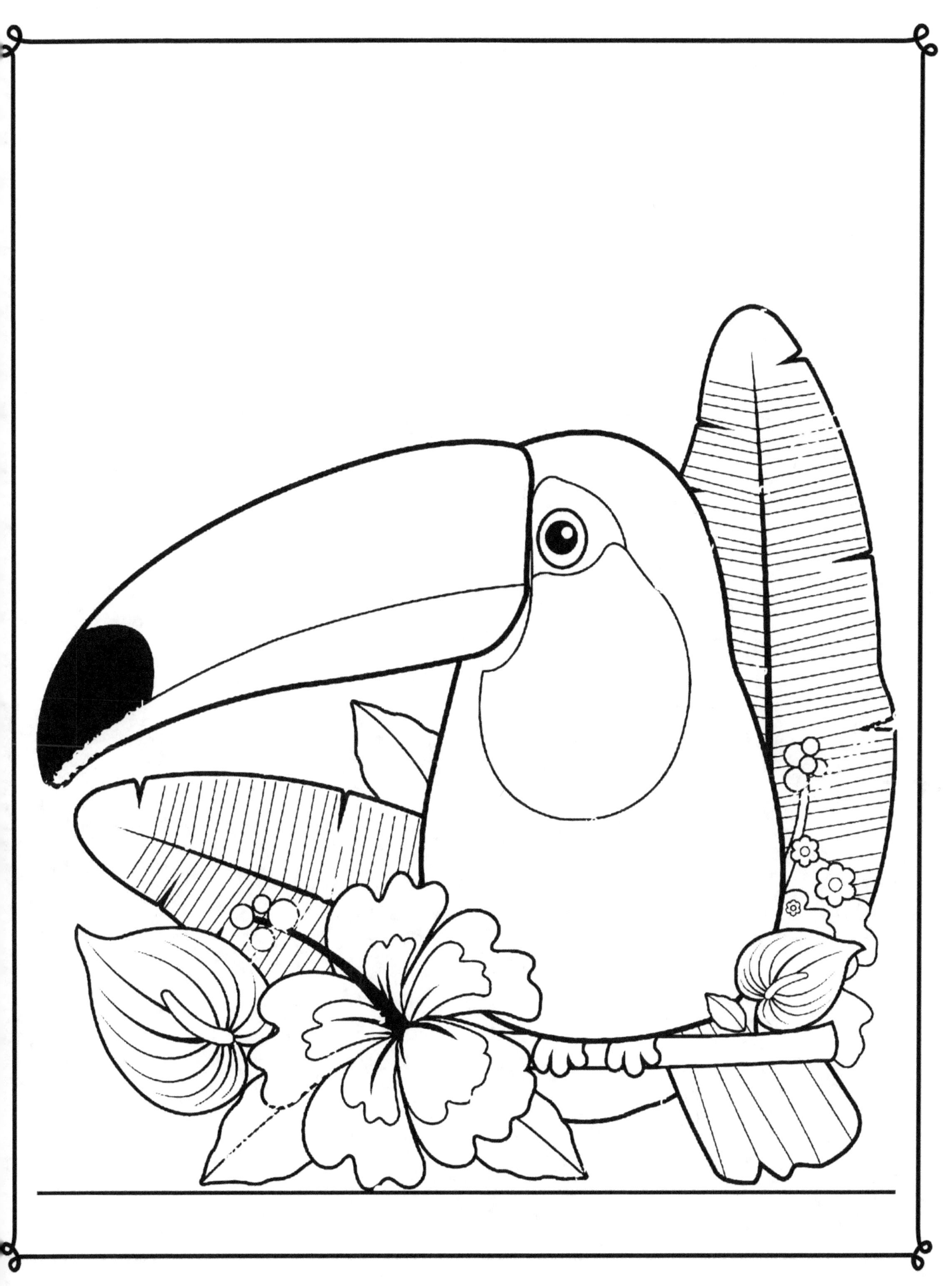

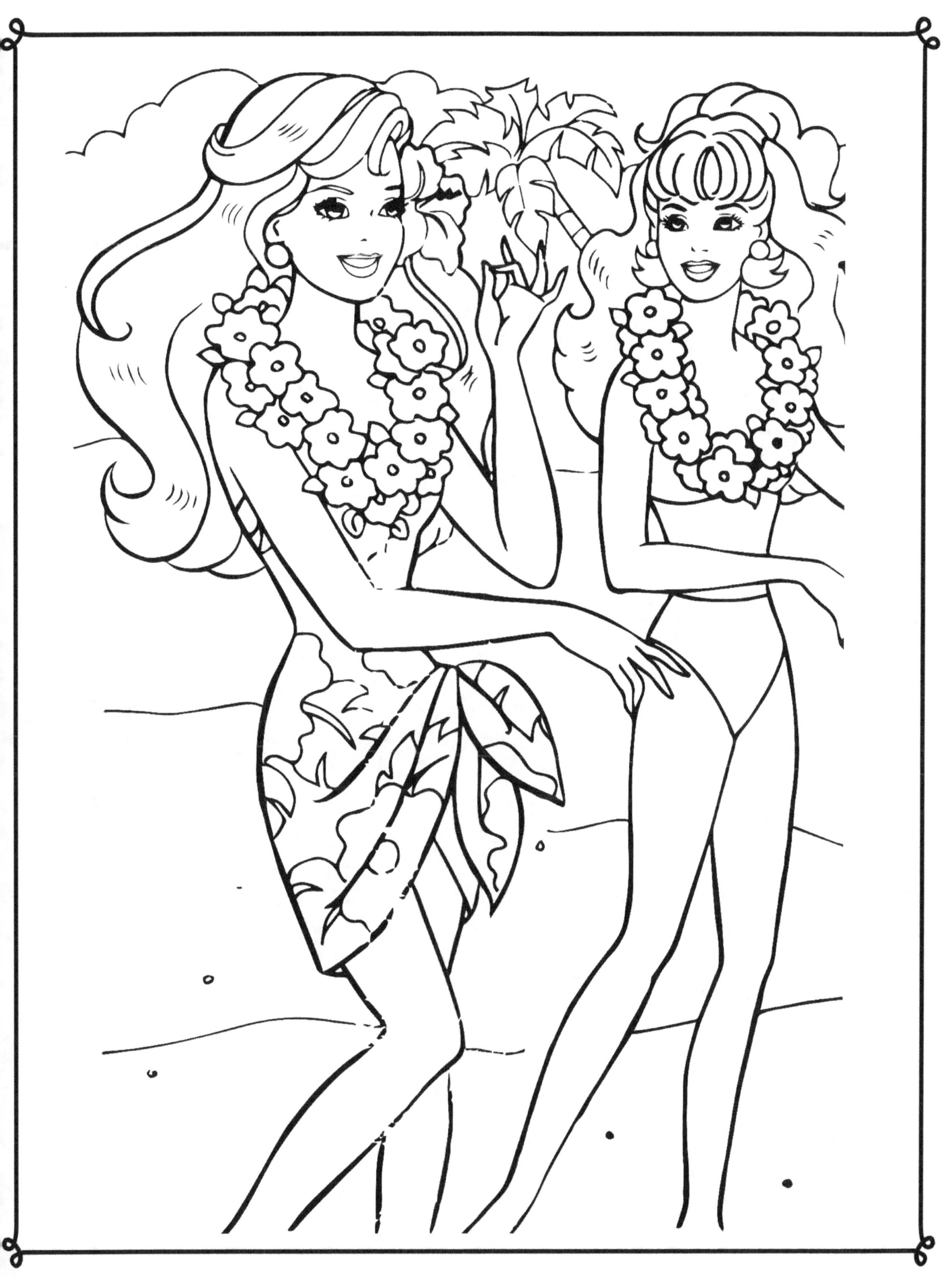

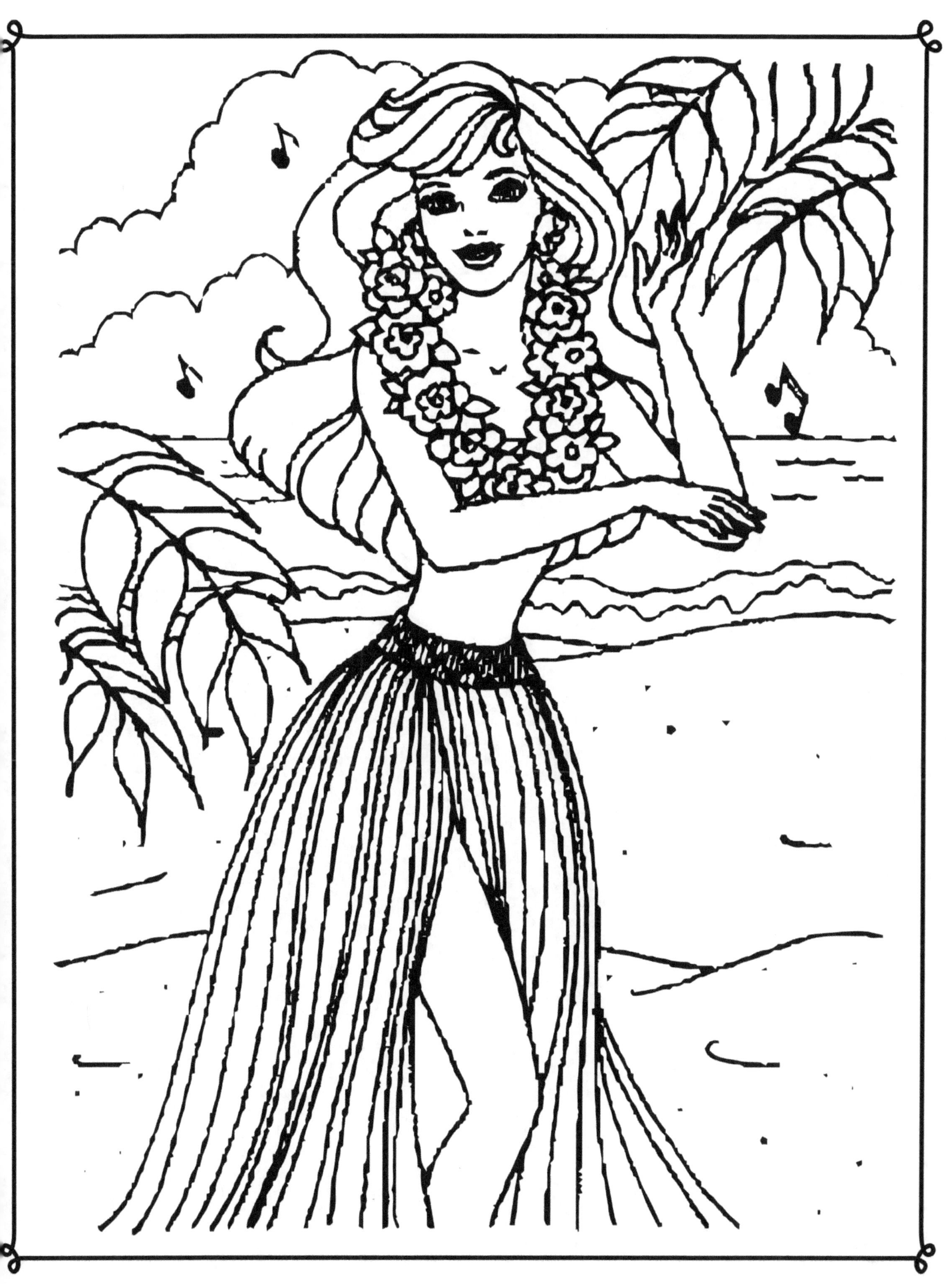

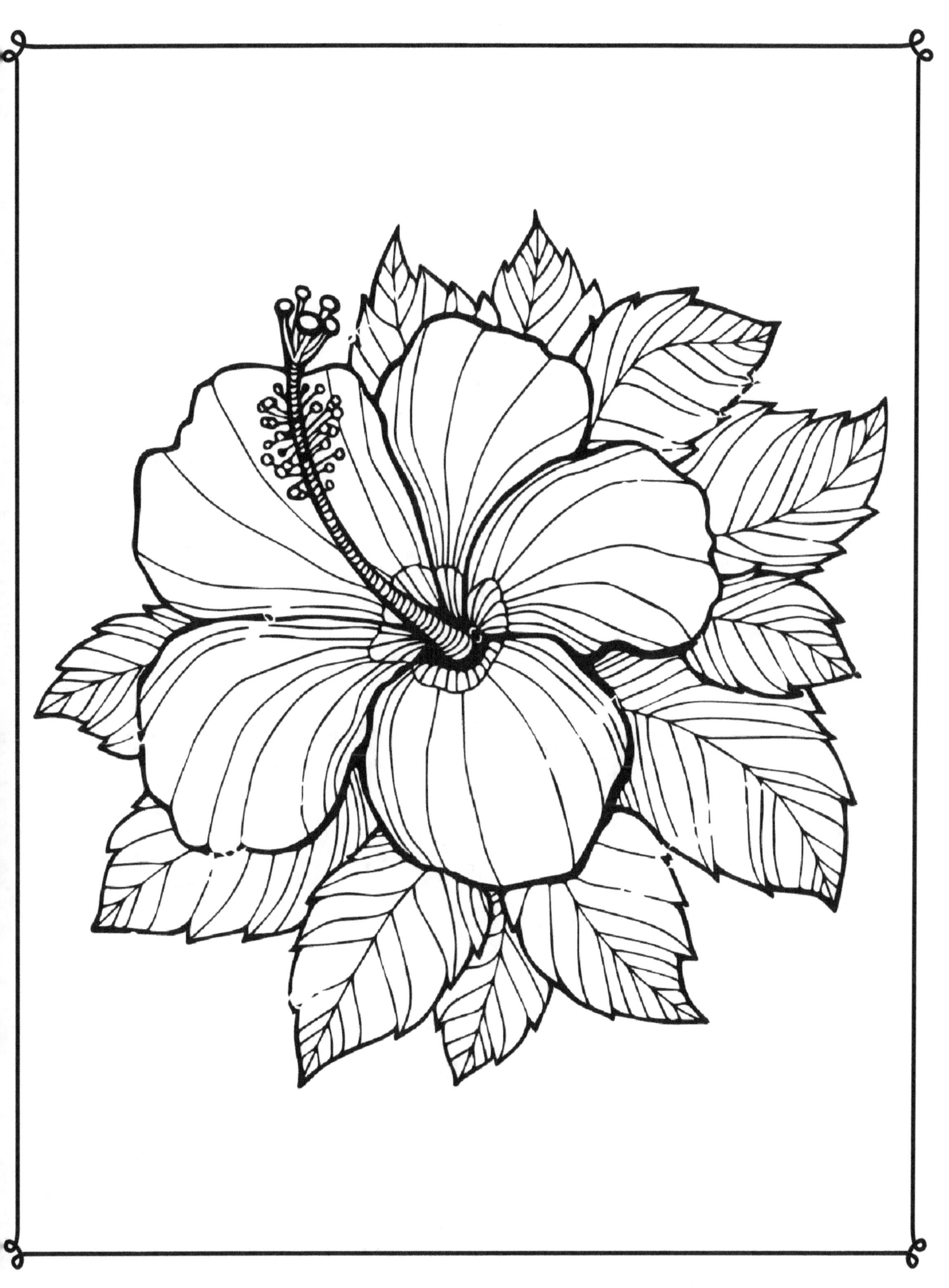

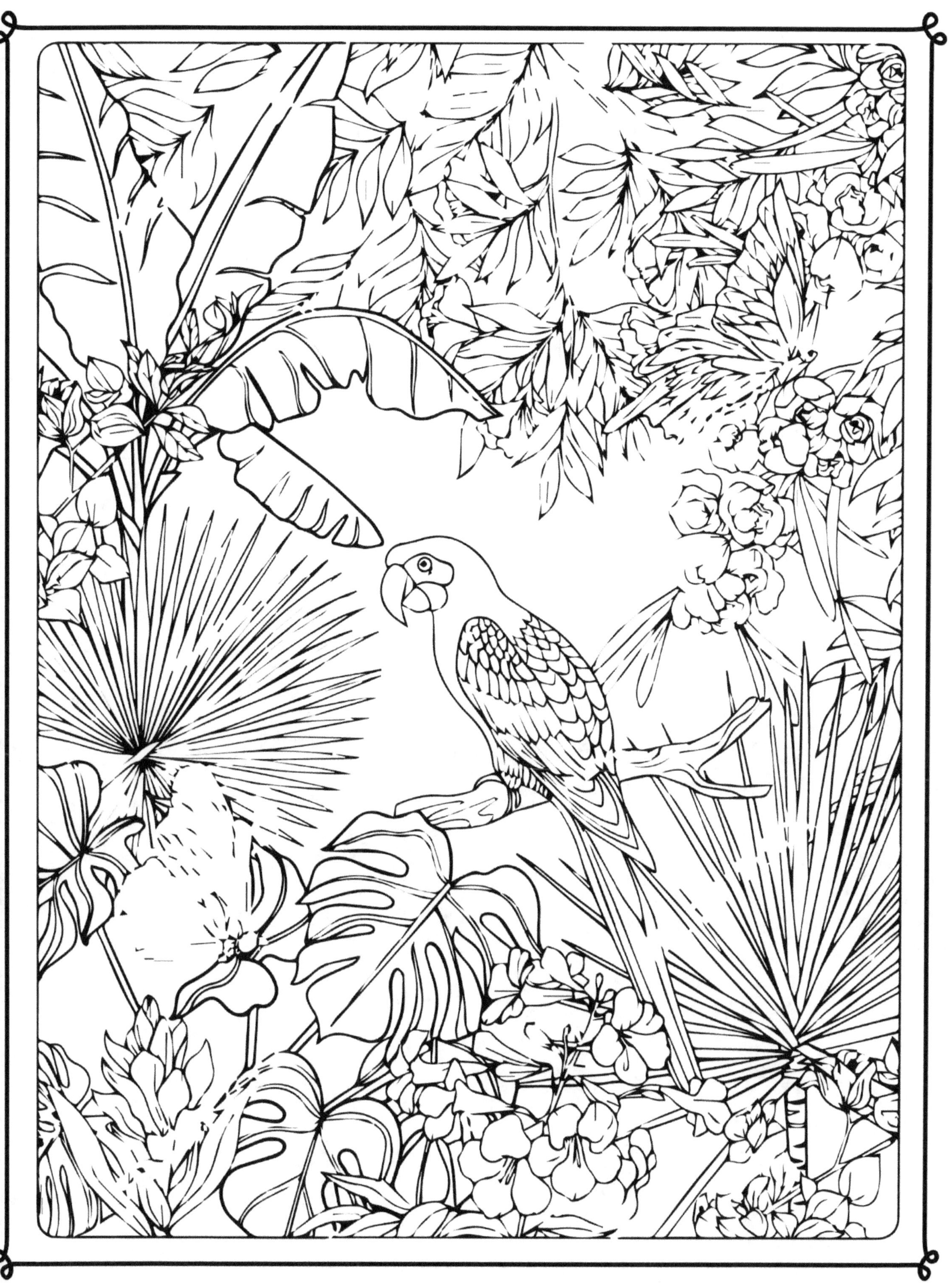

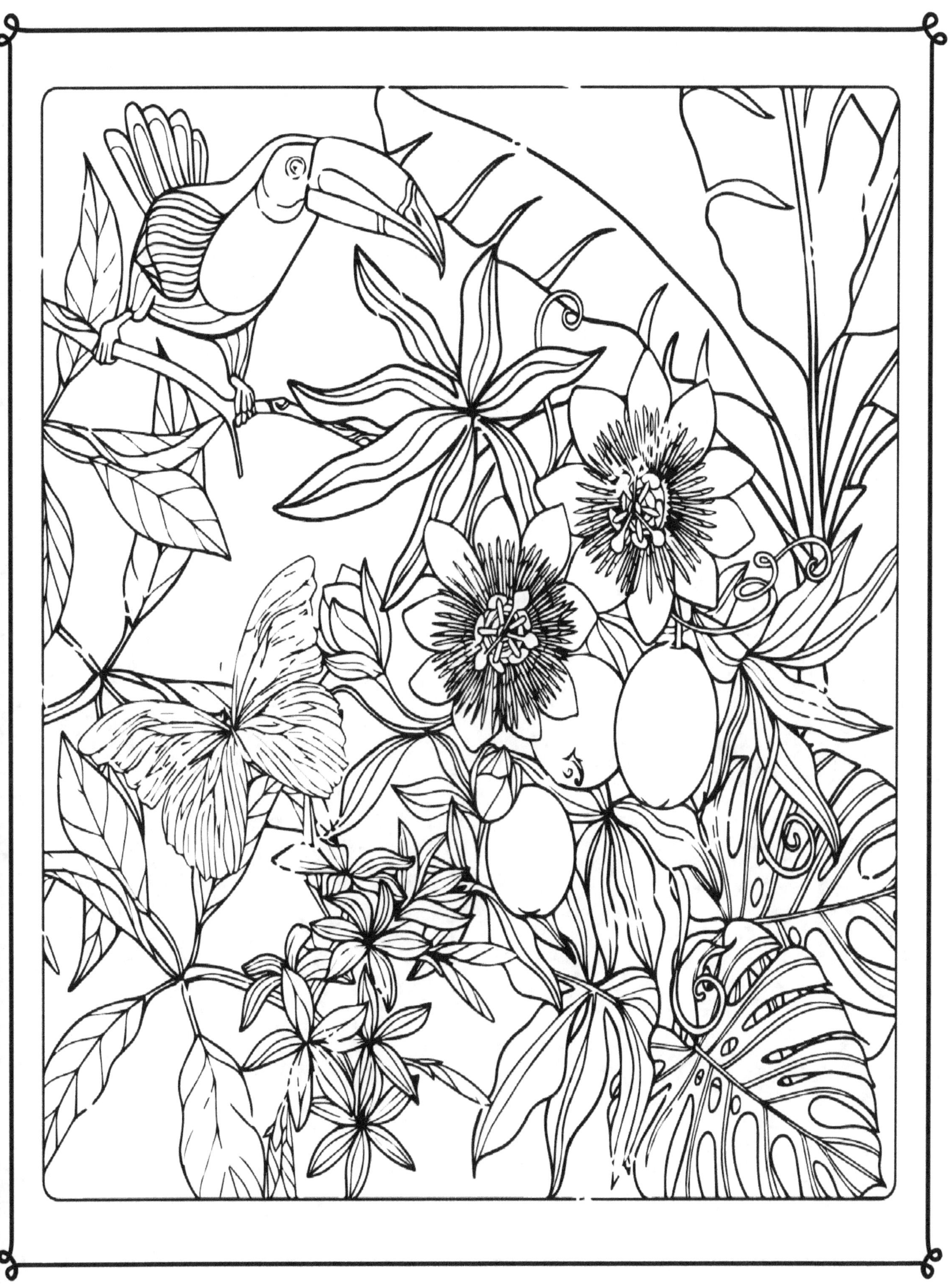

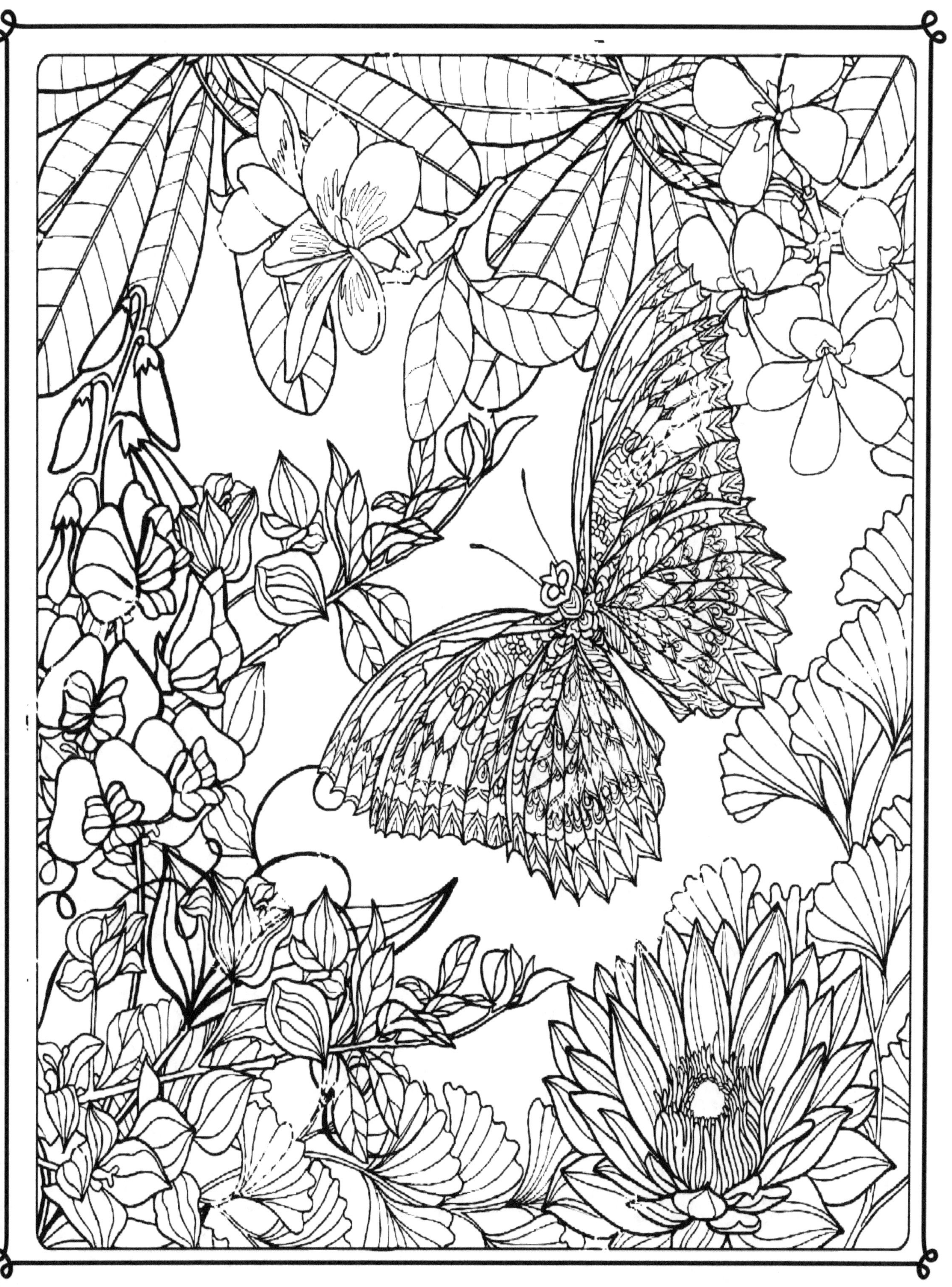

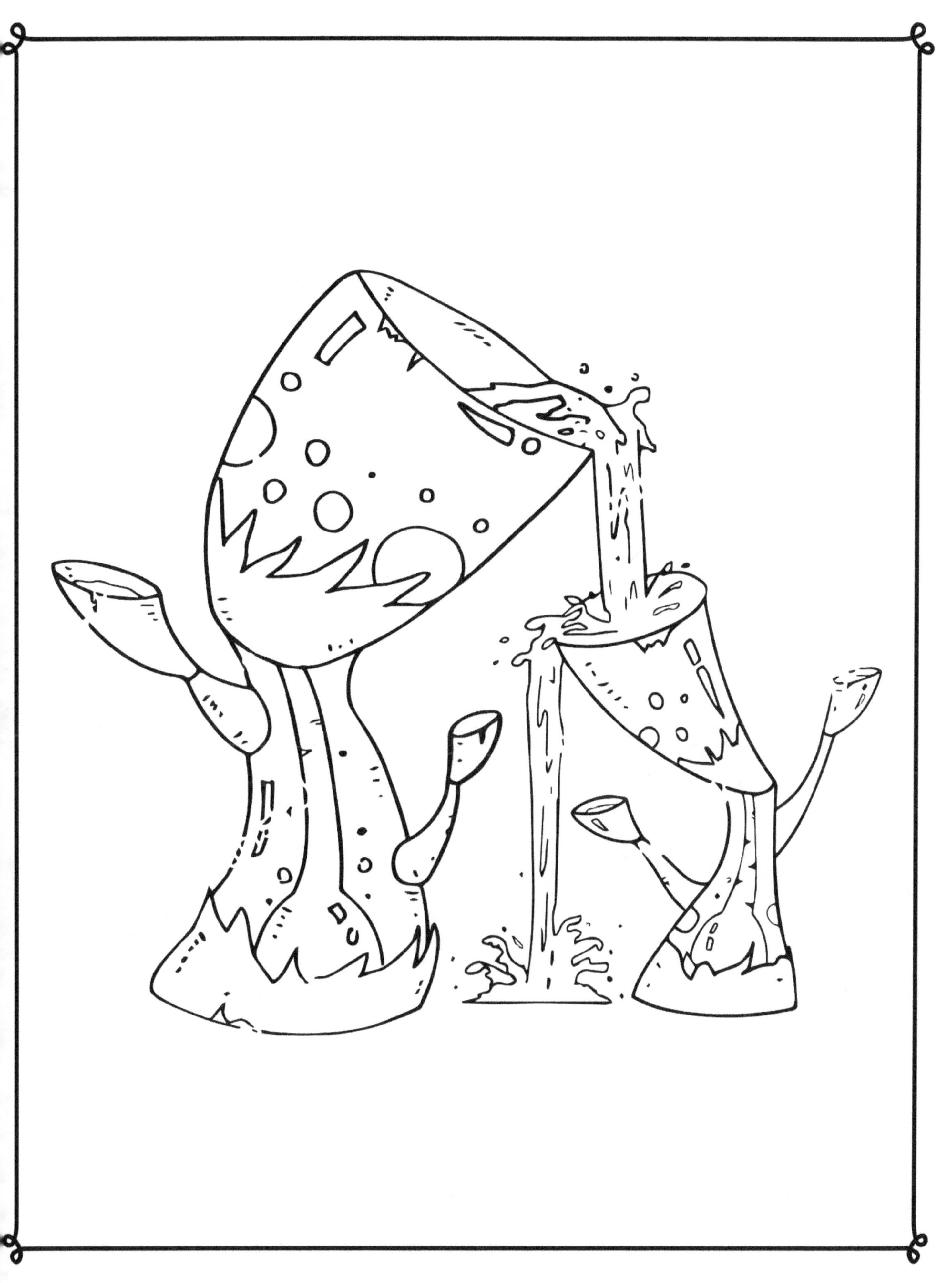

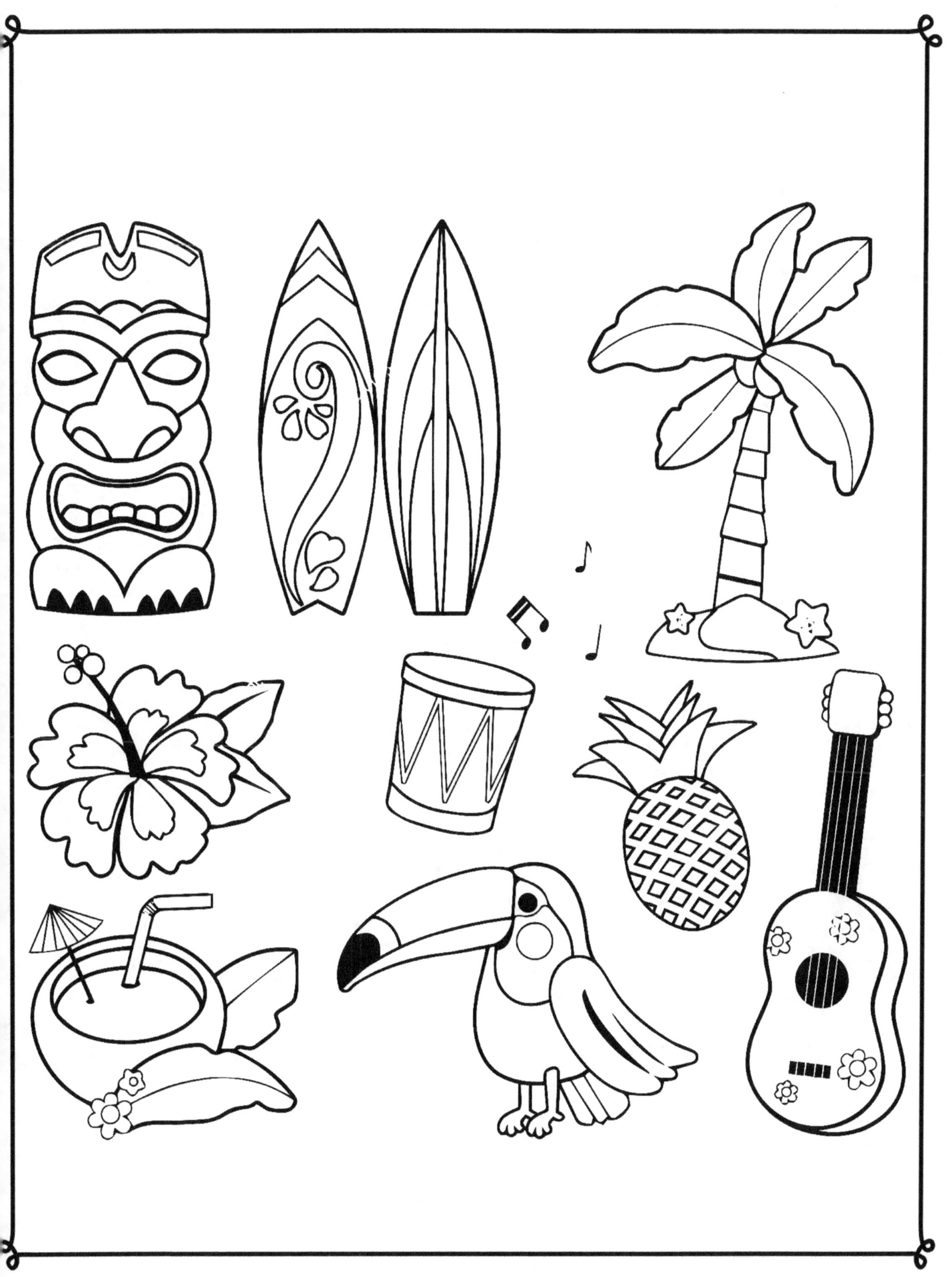

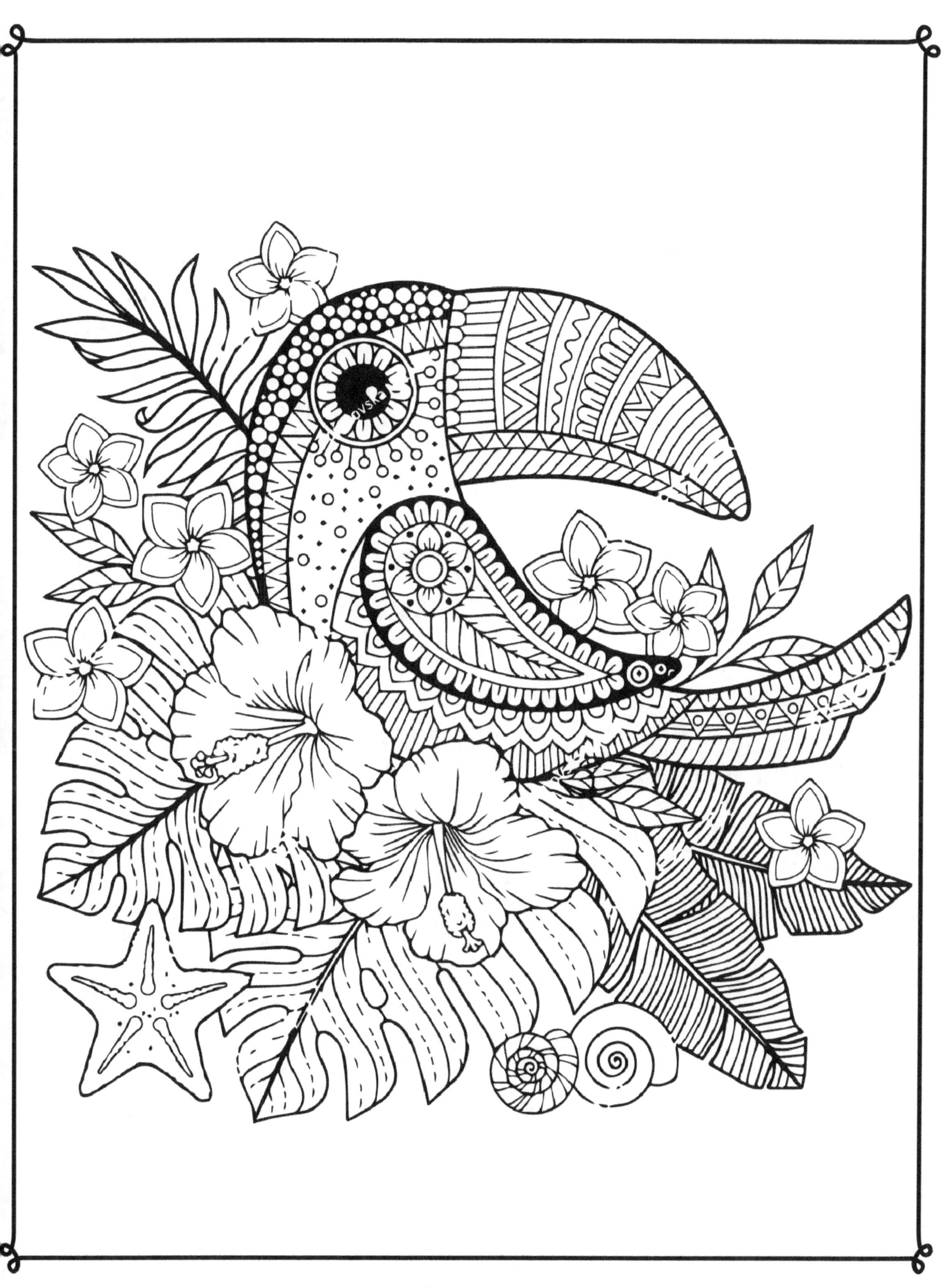

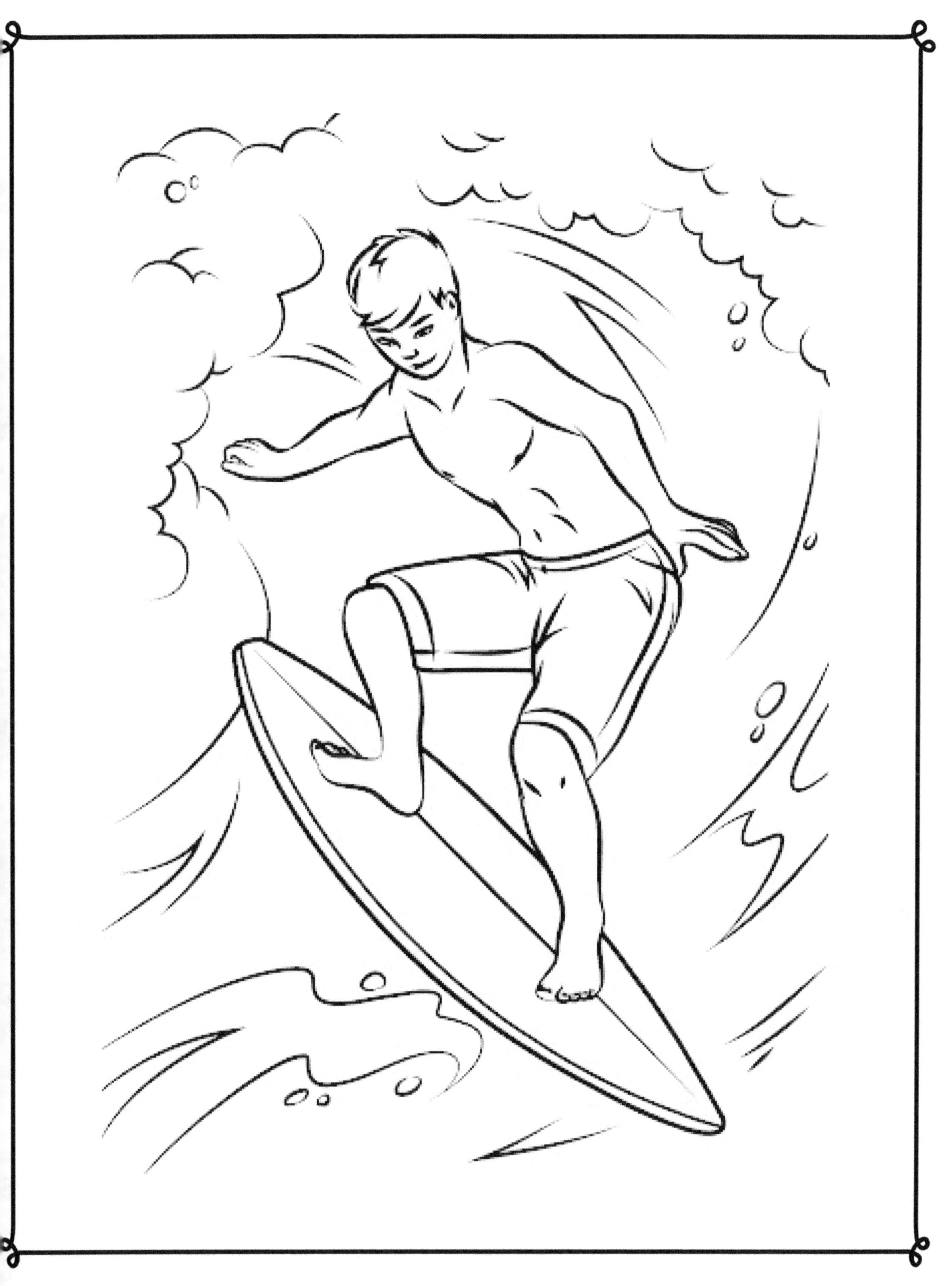

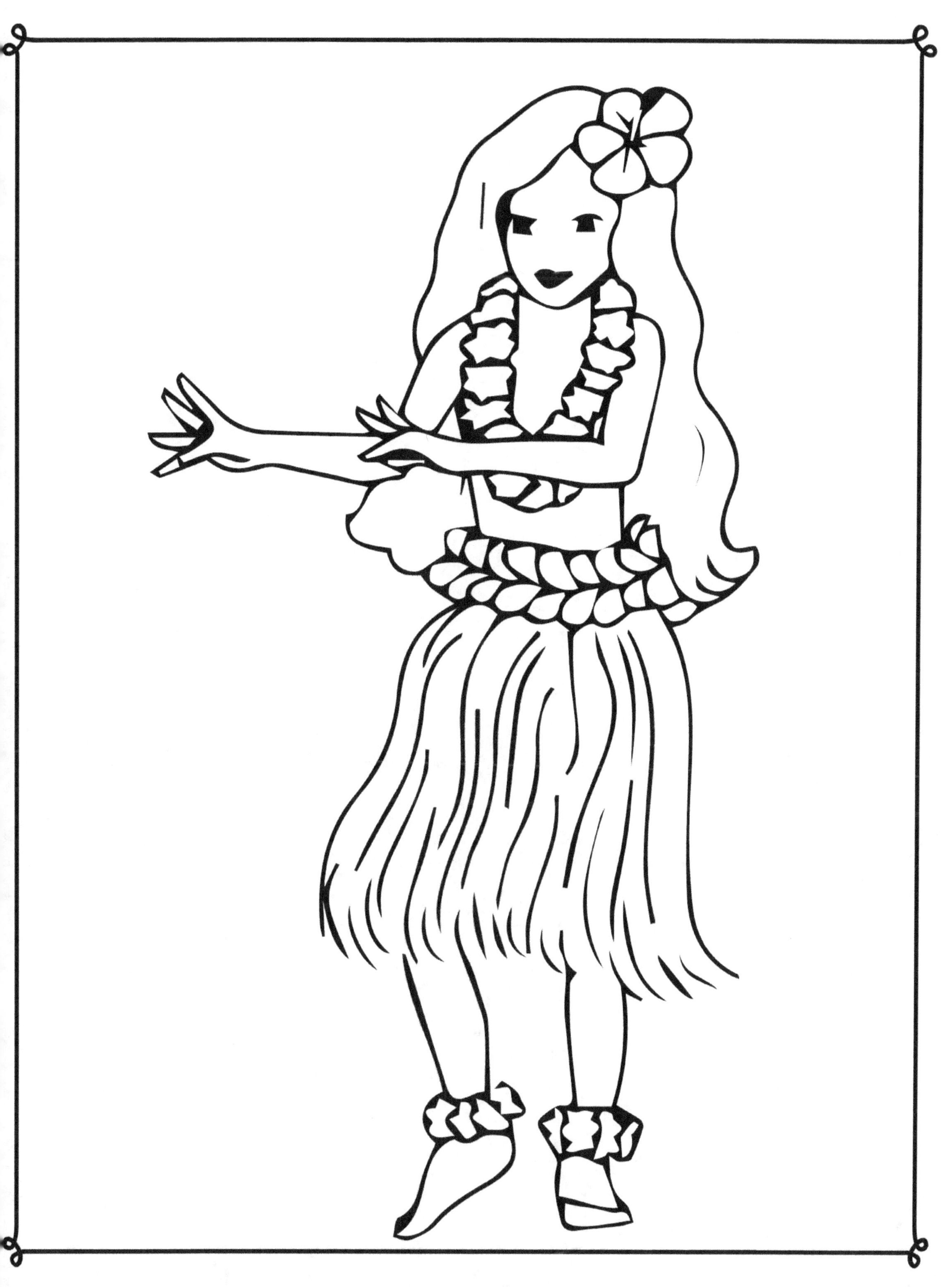

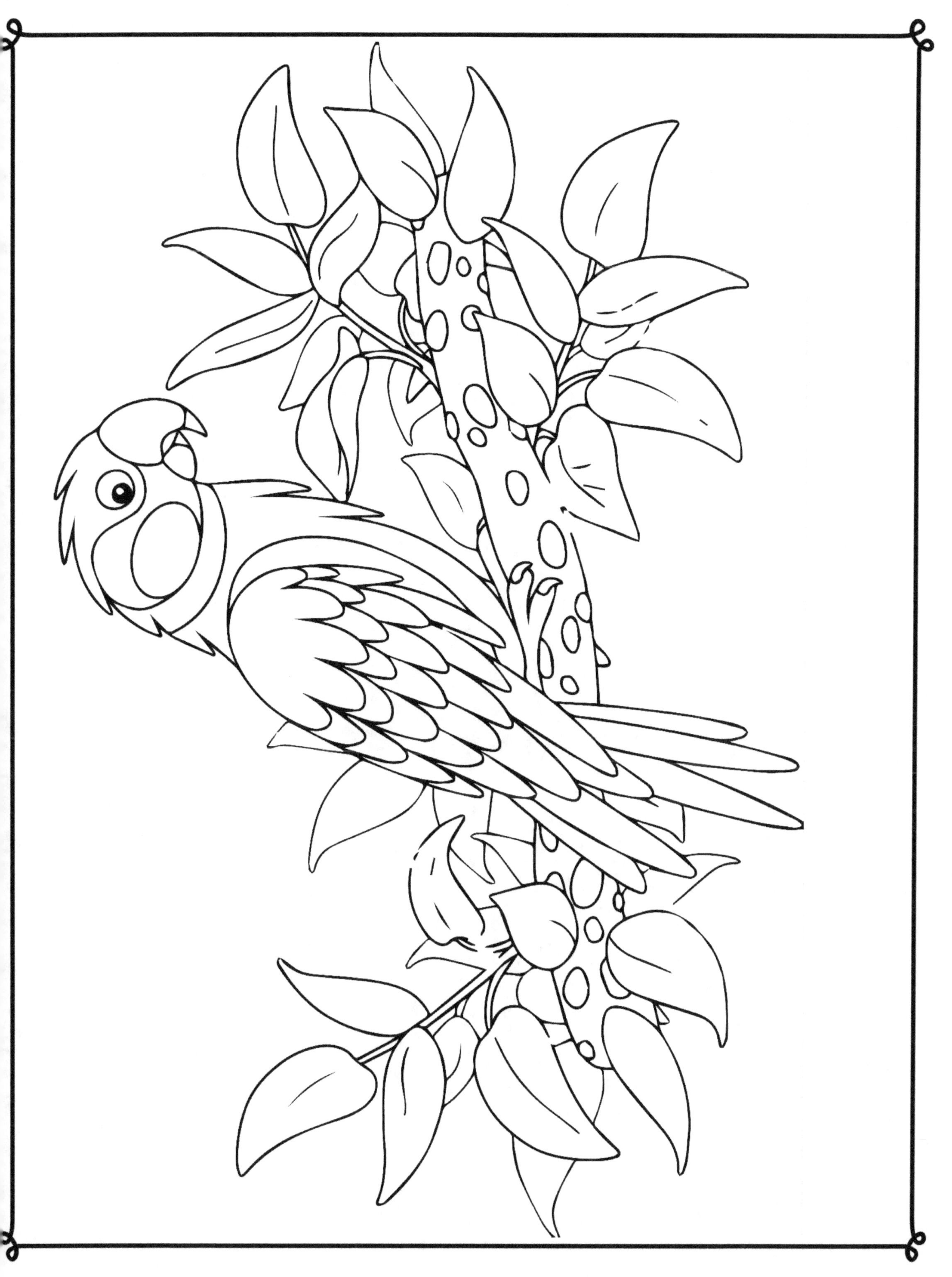

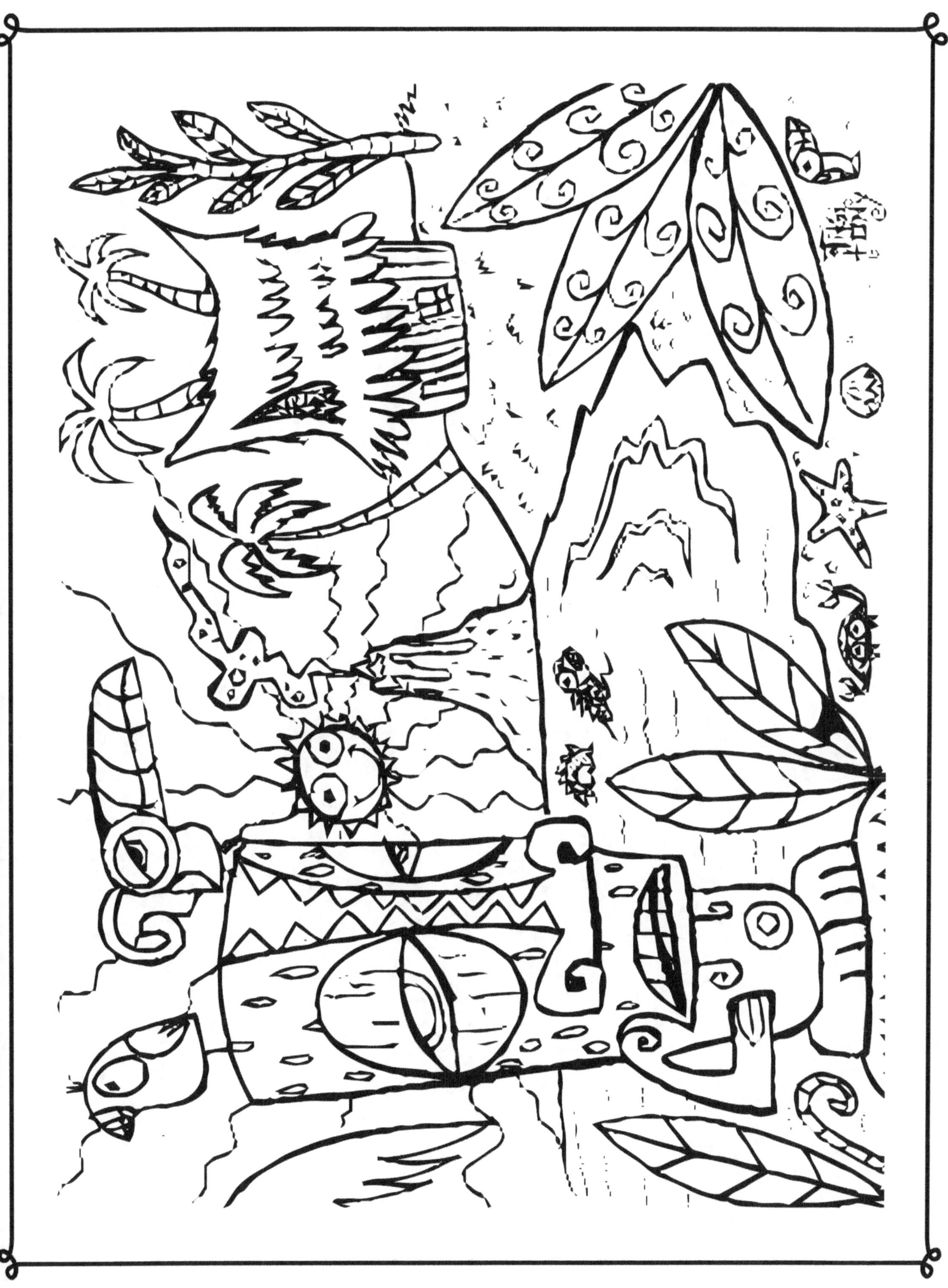

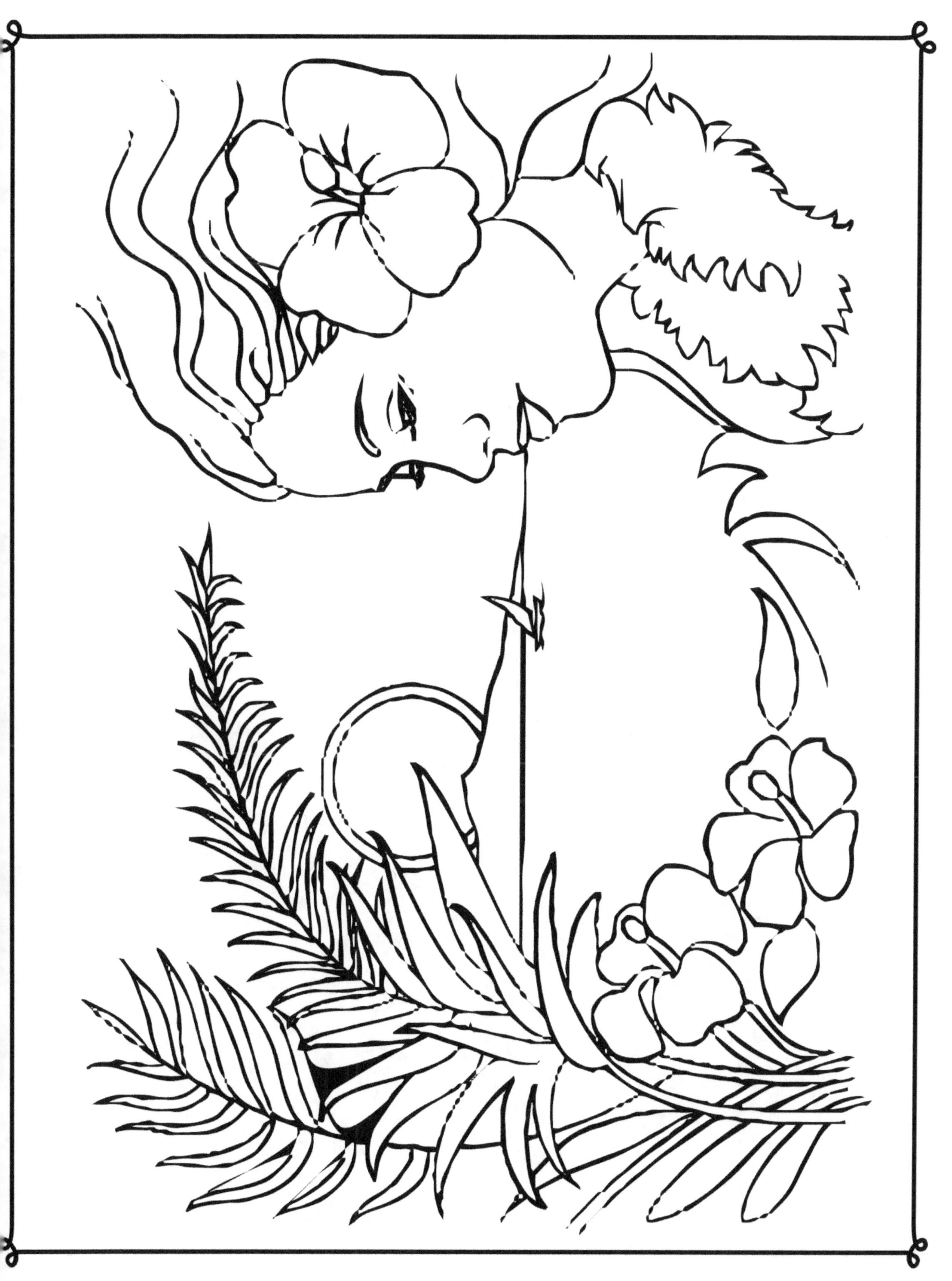

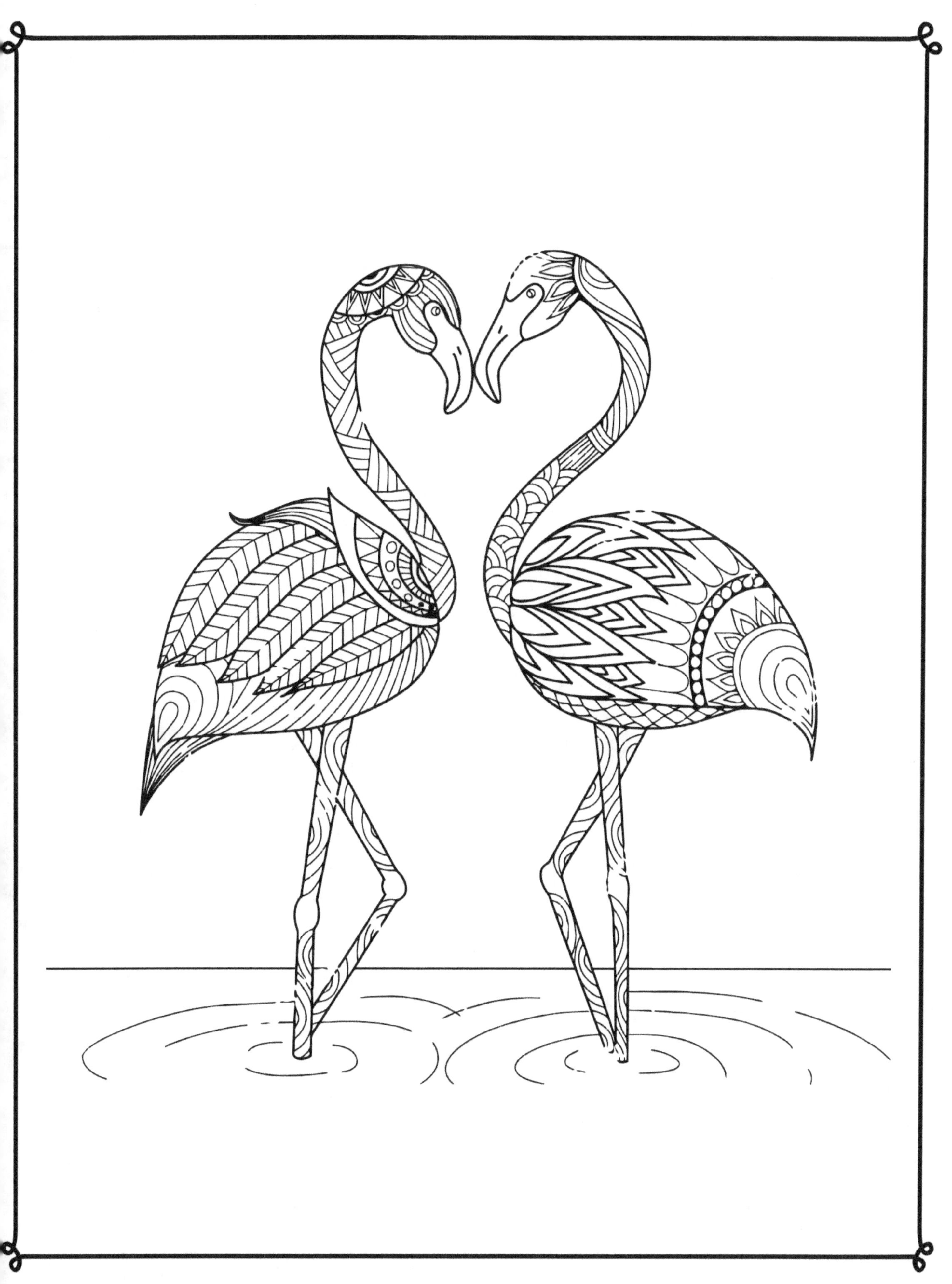

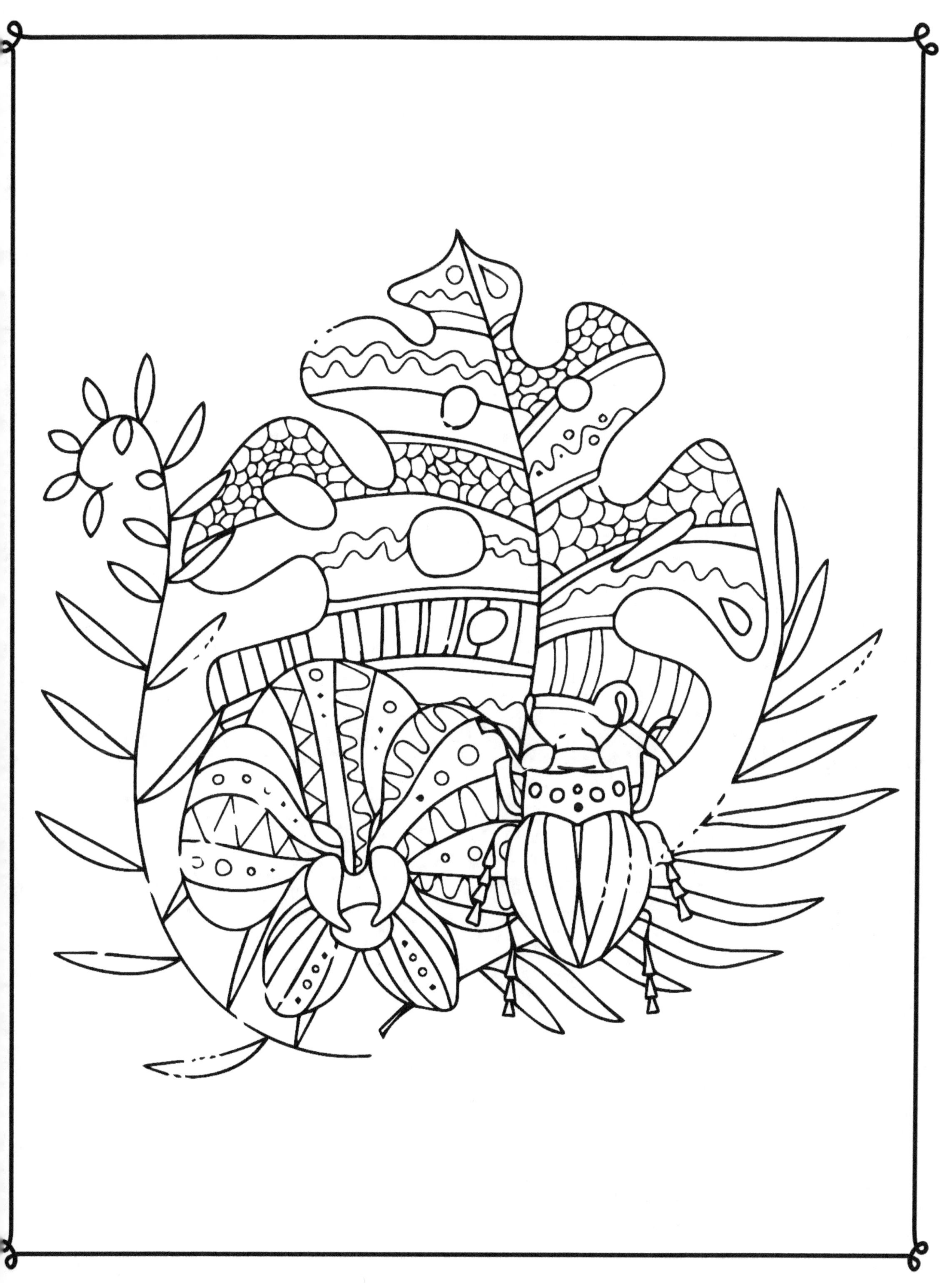

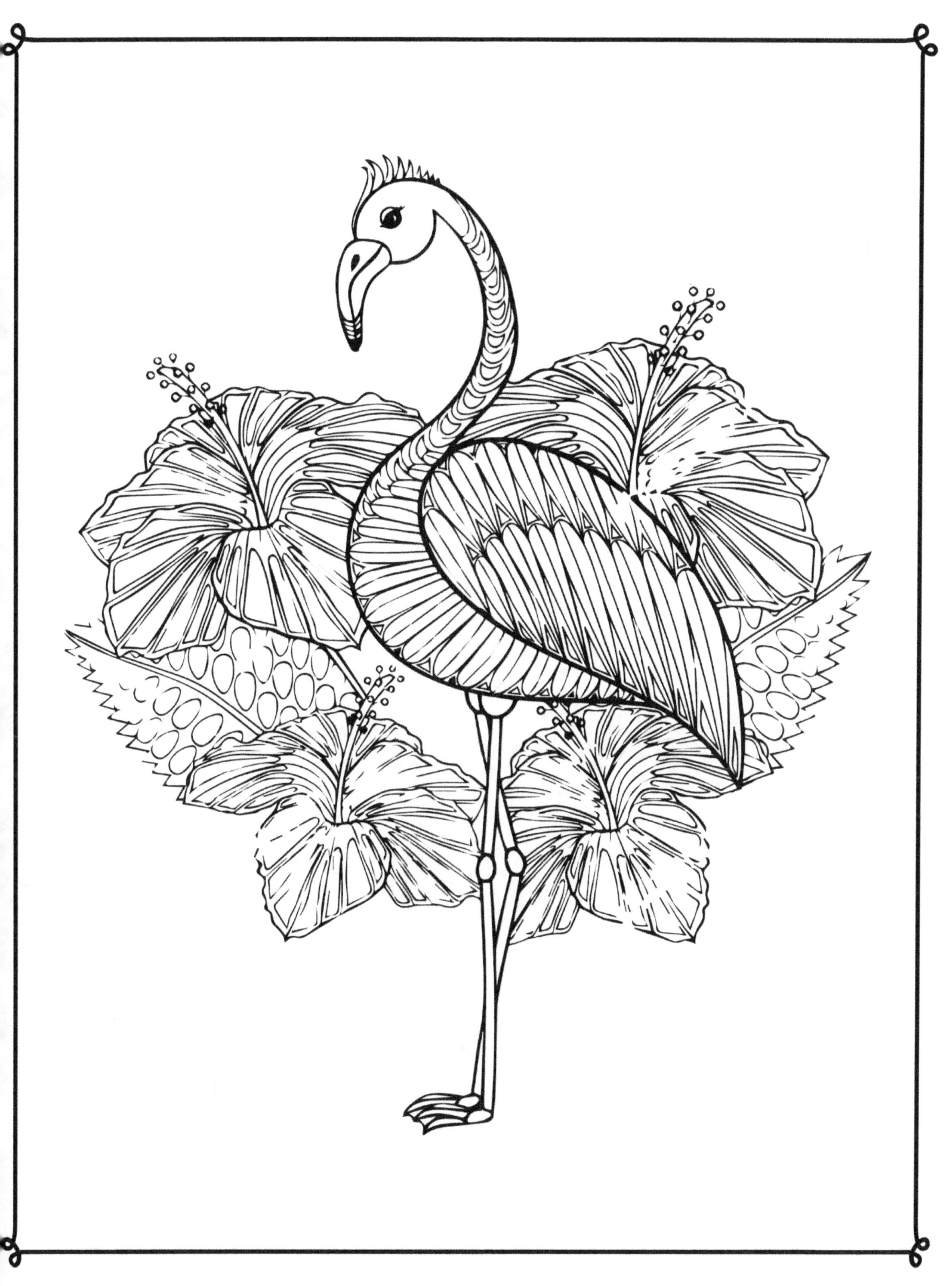

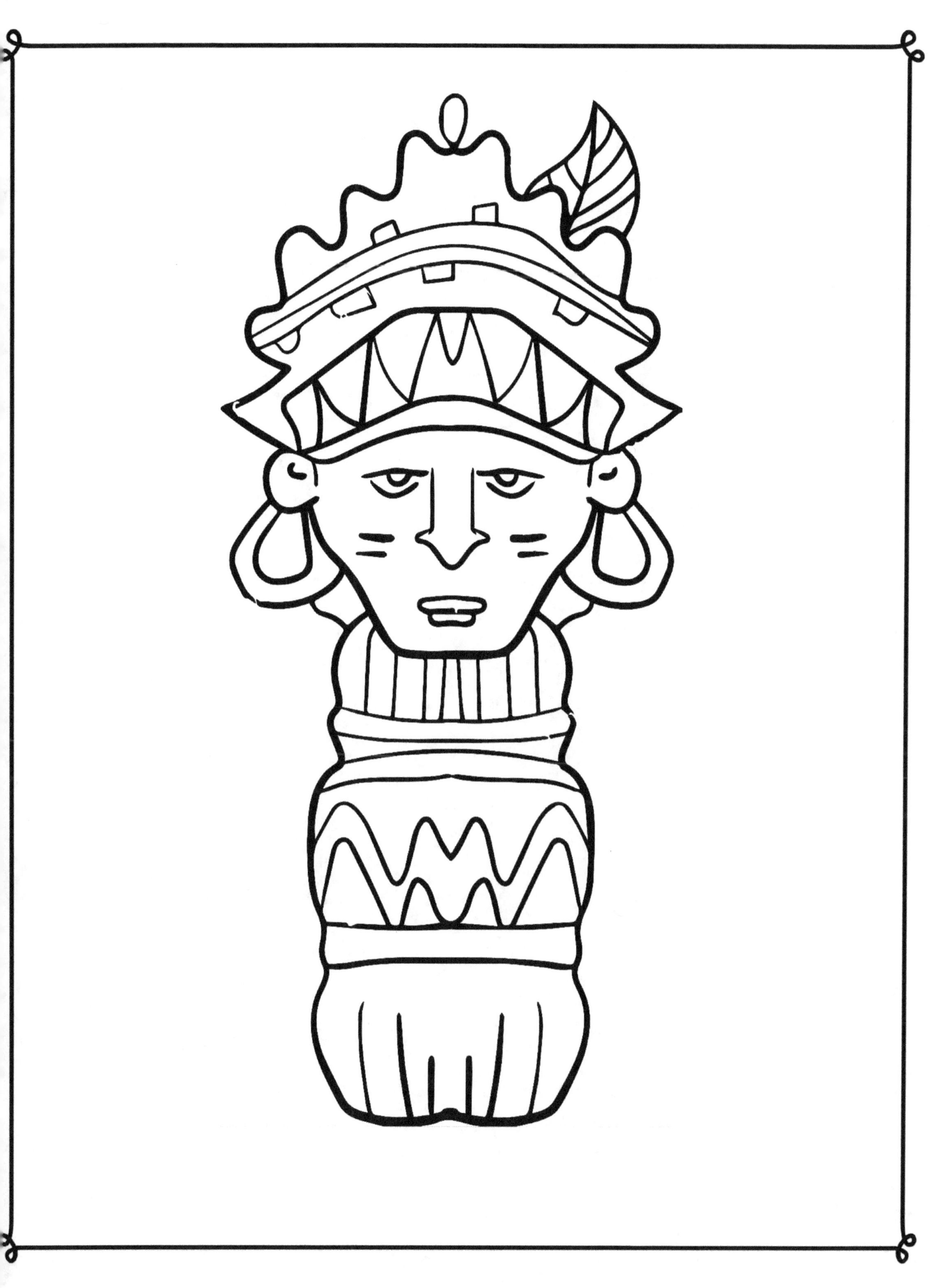

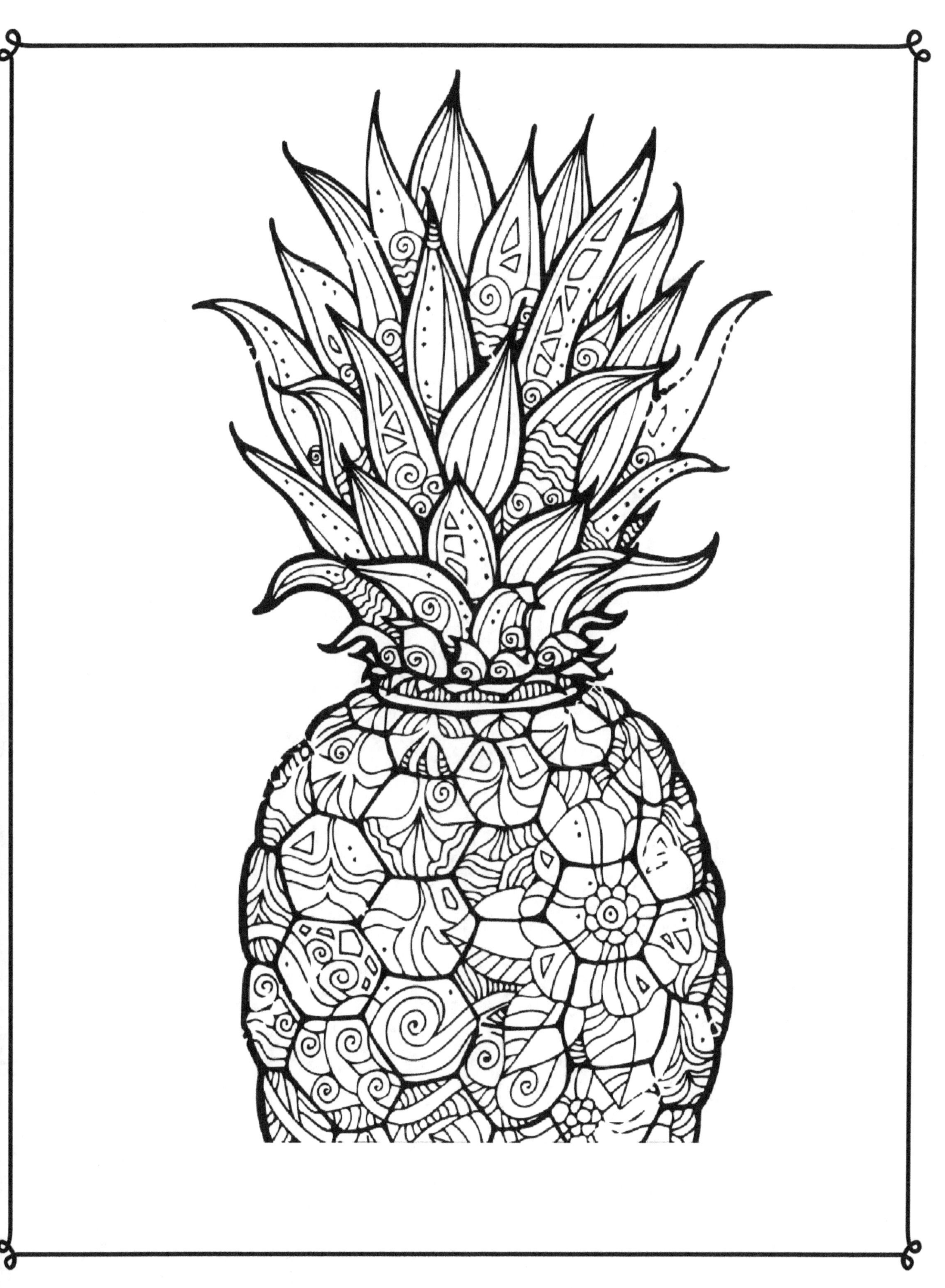

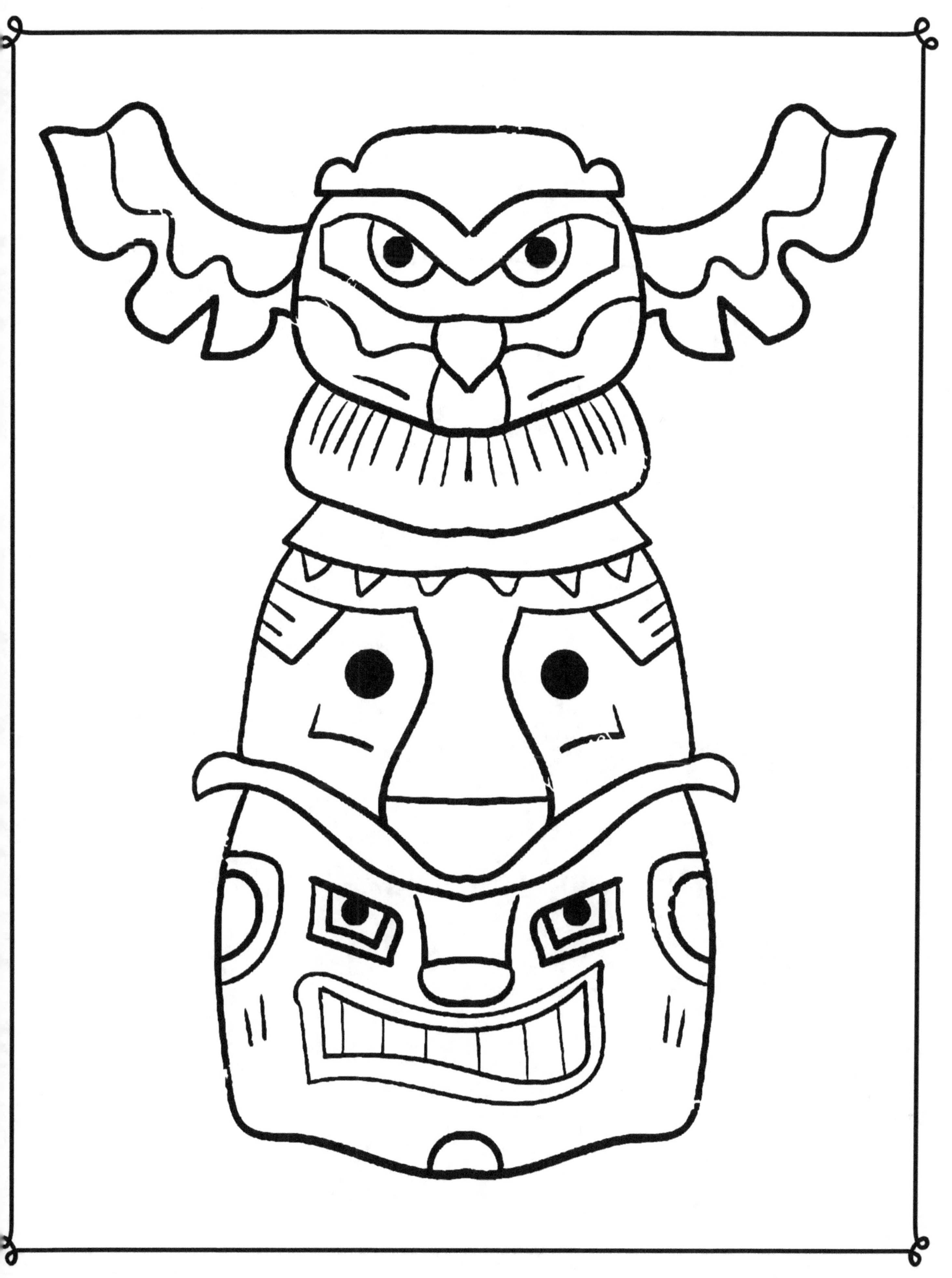

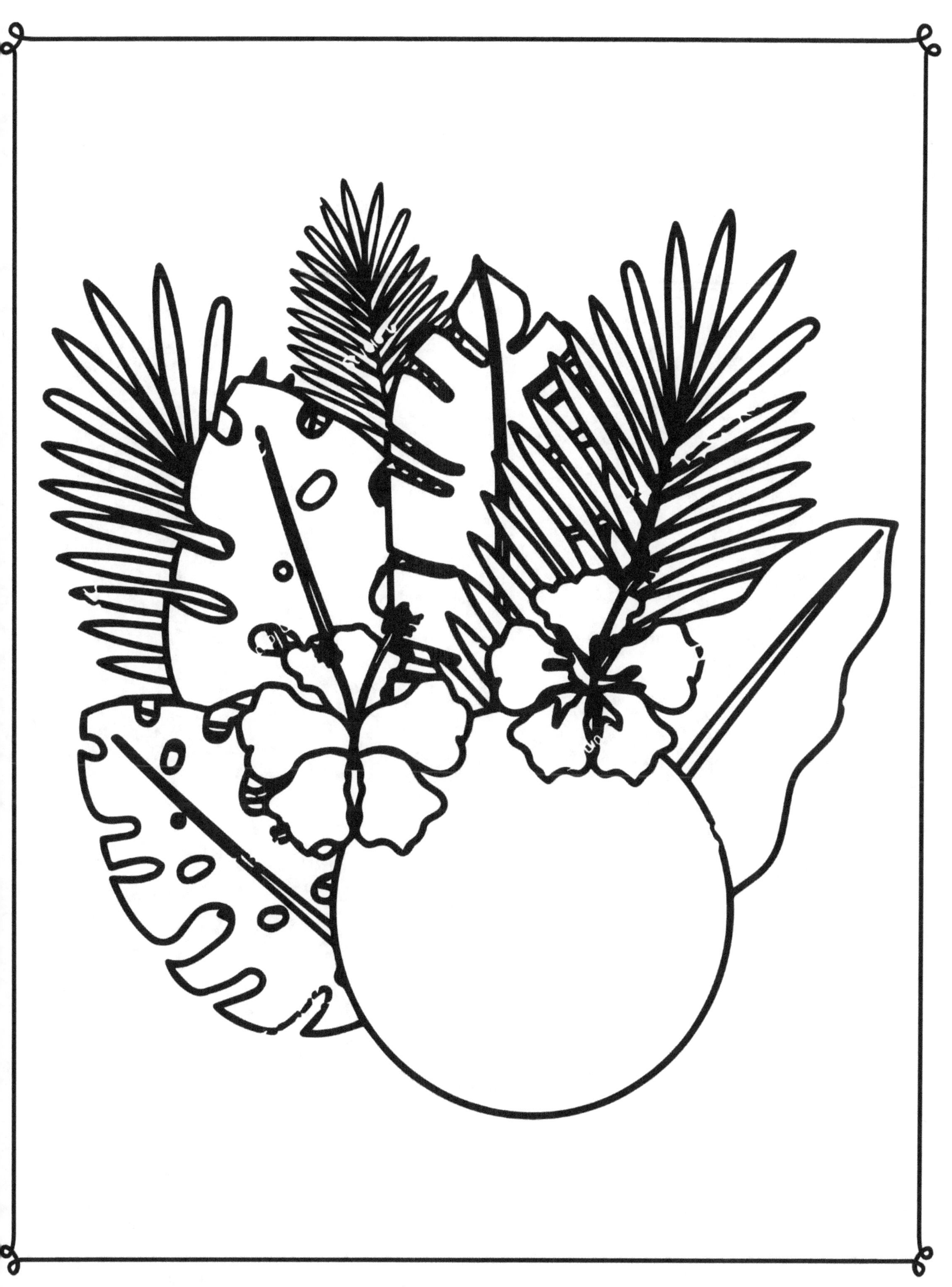

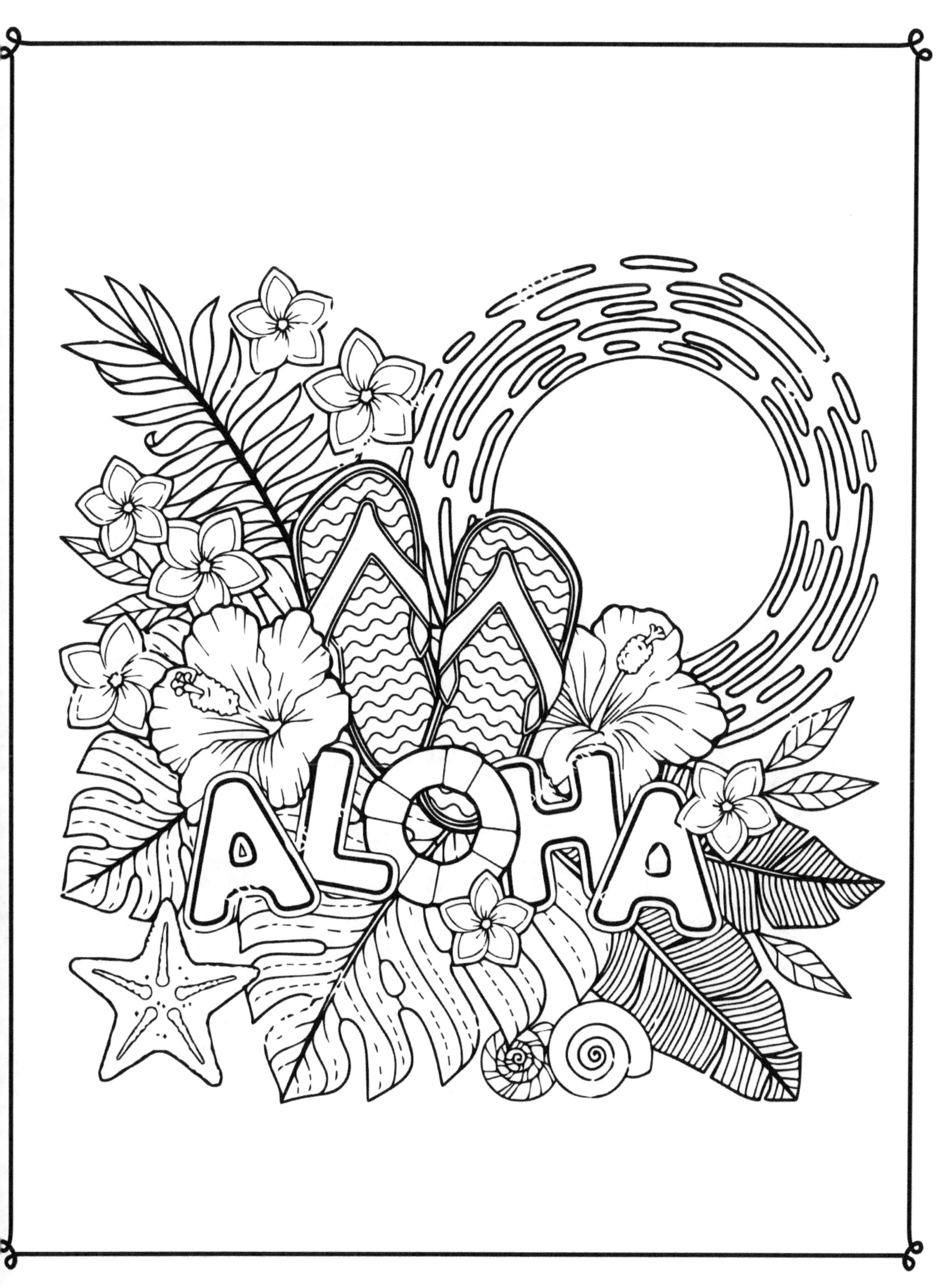
ALOHA

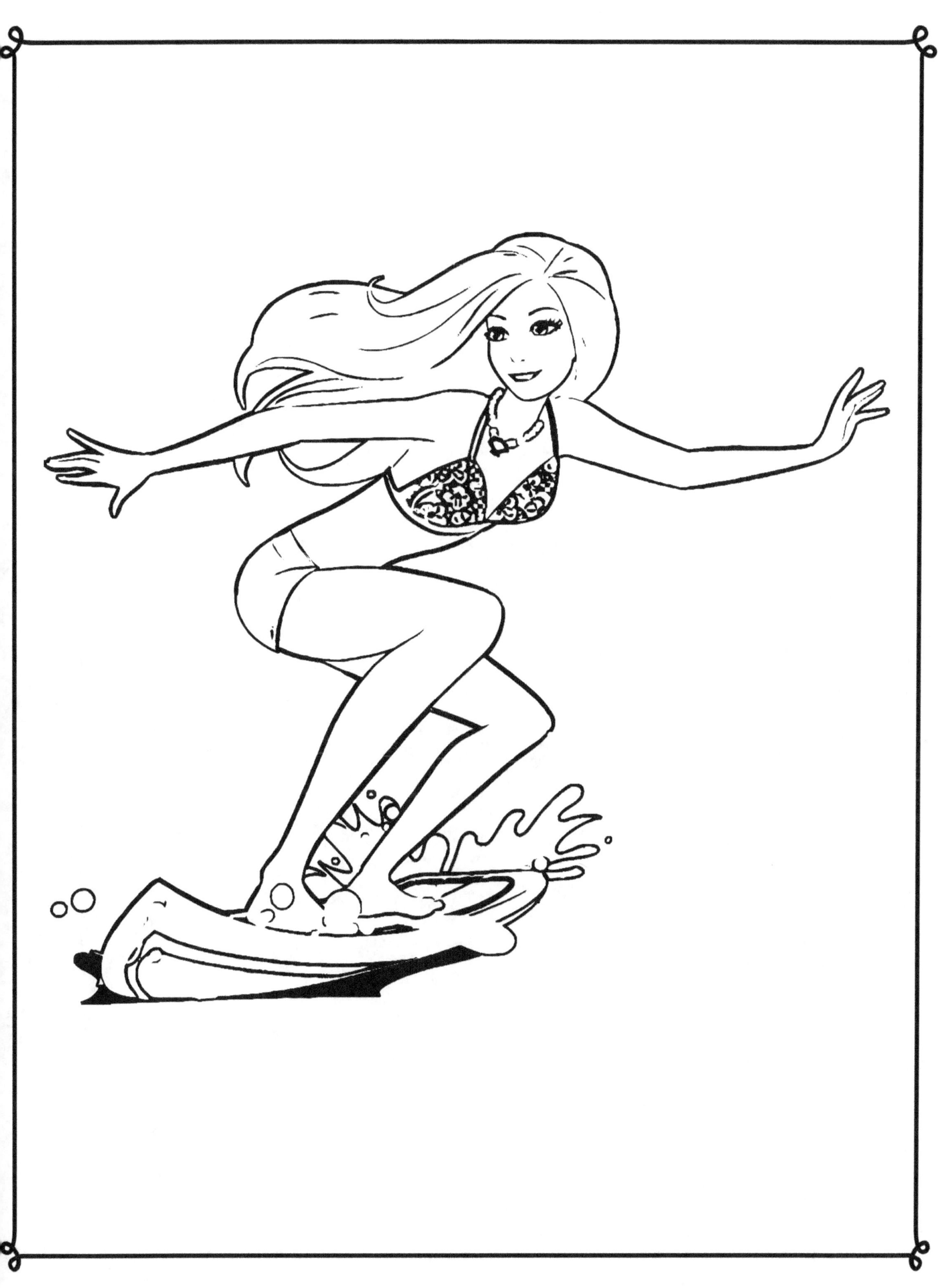

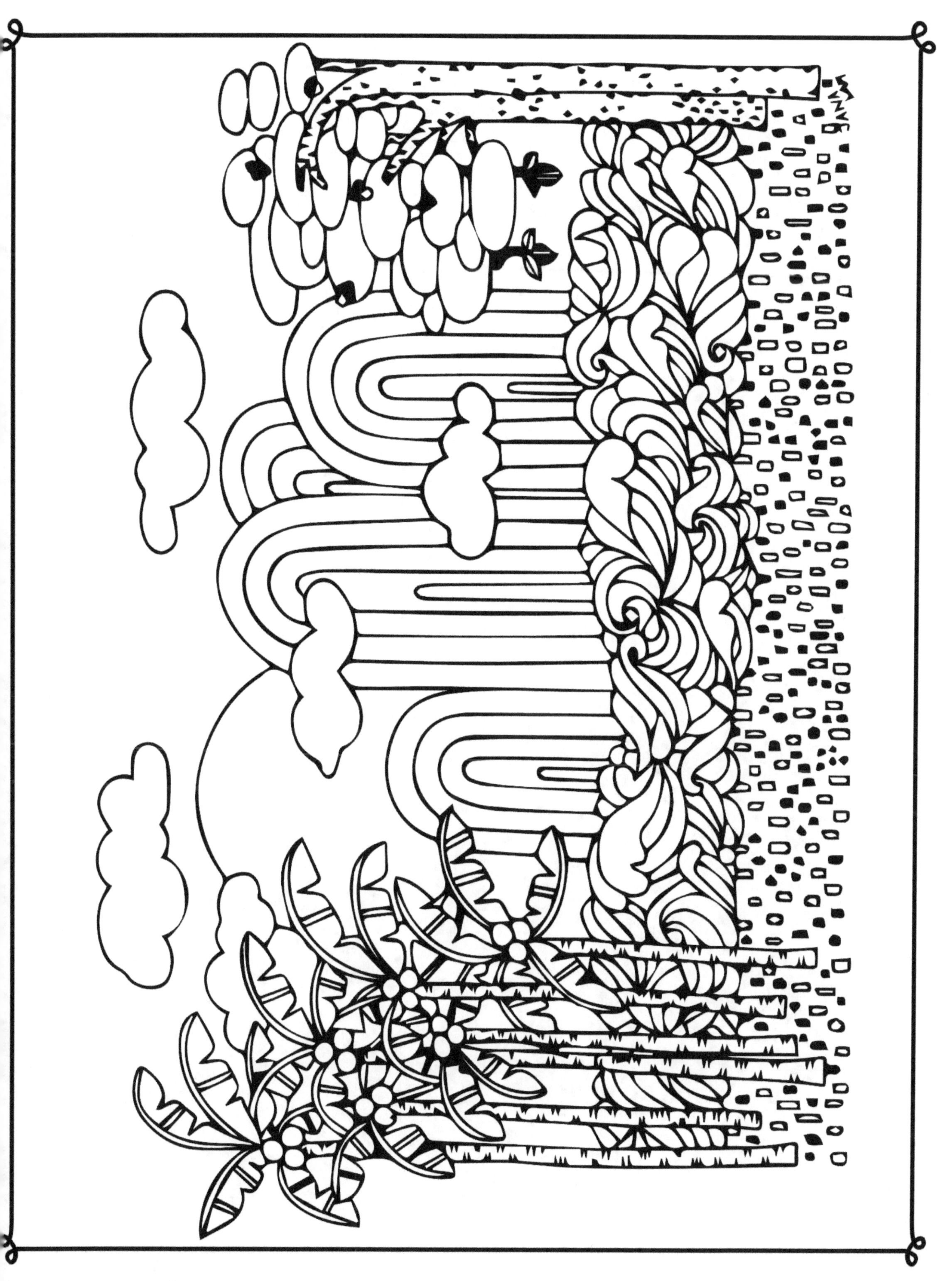

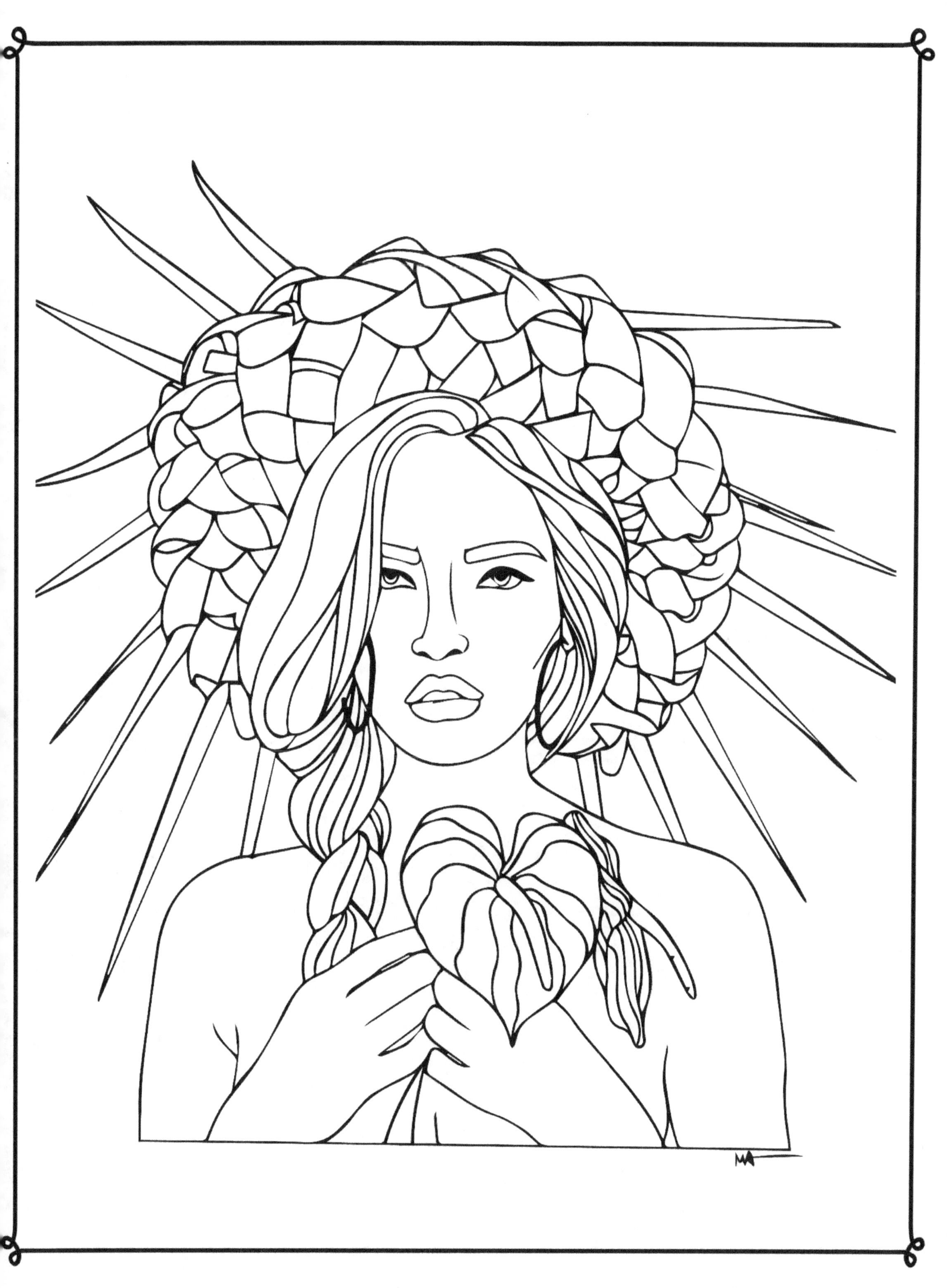

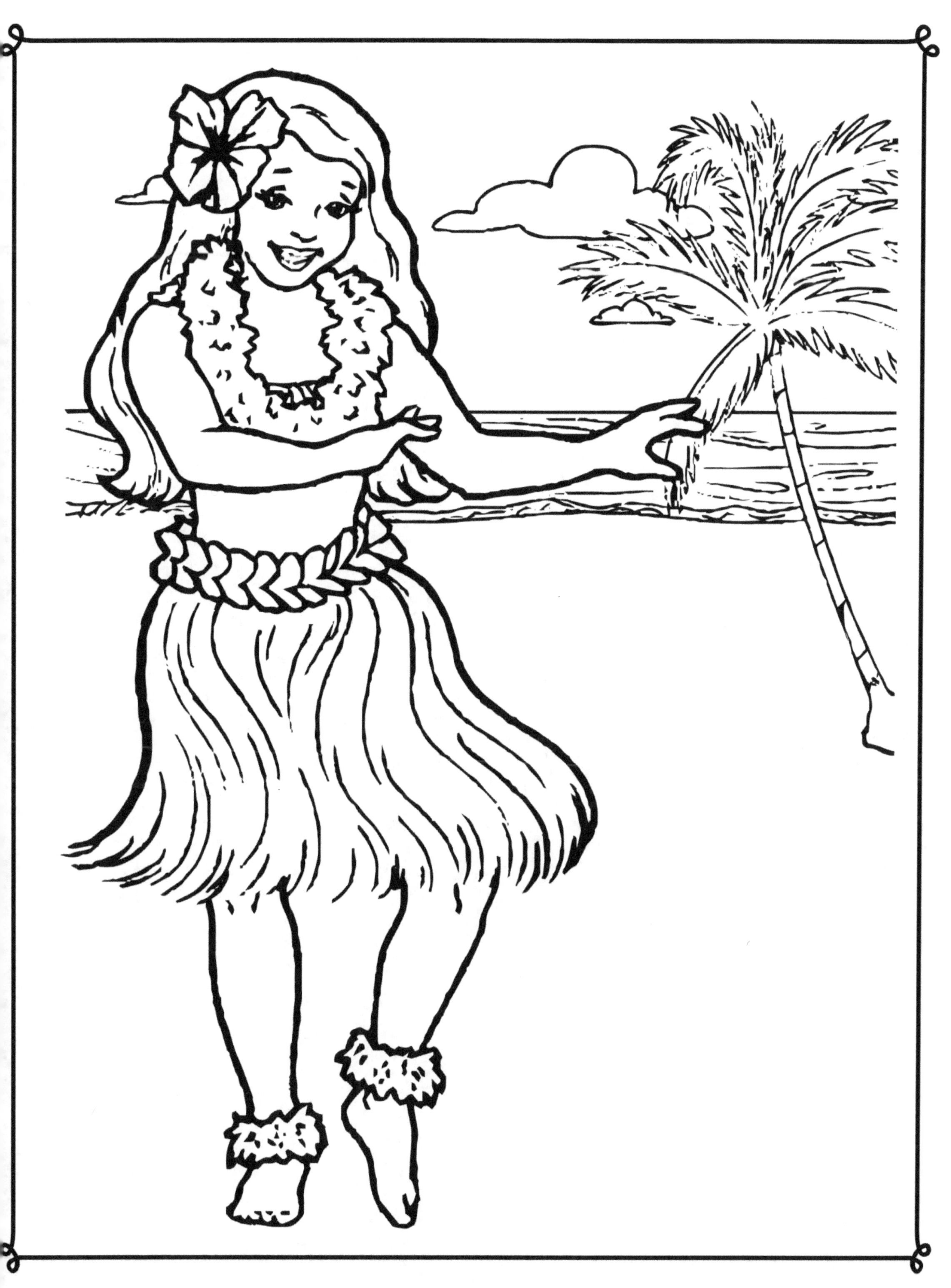

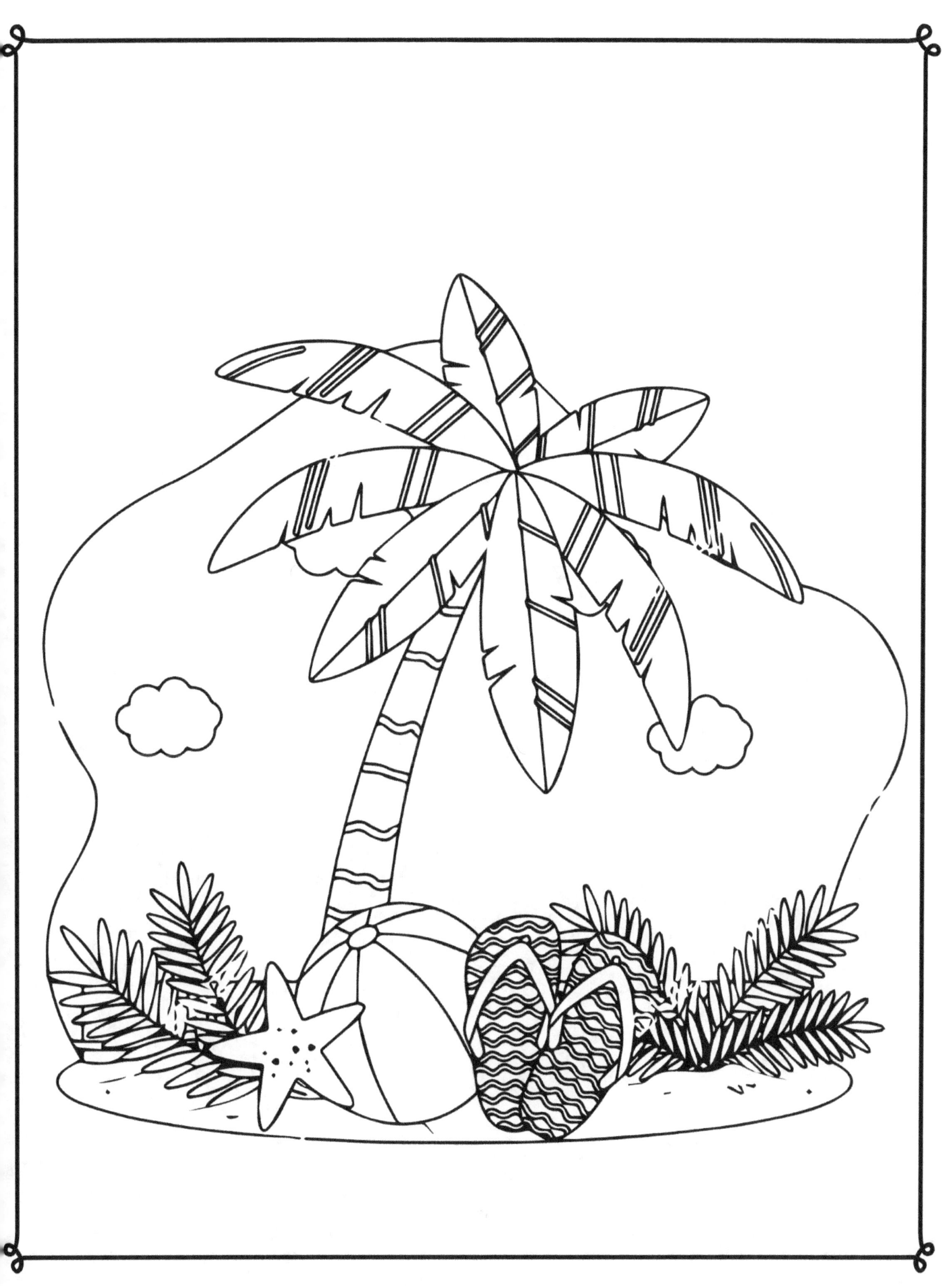

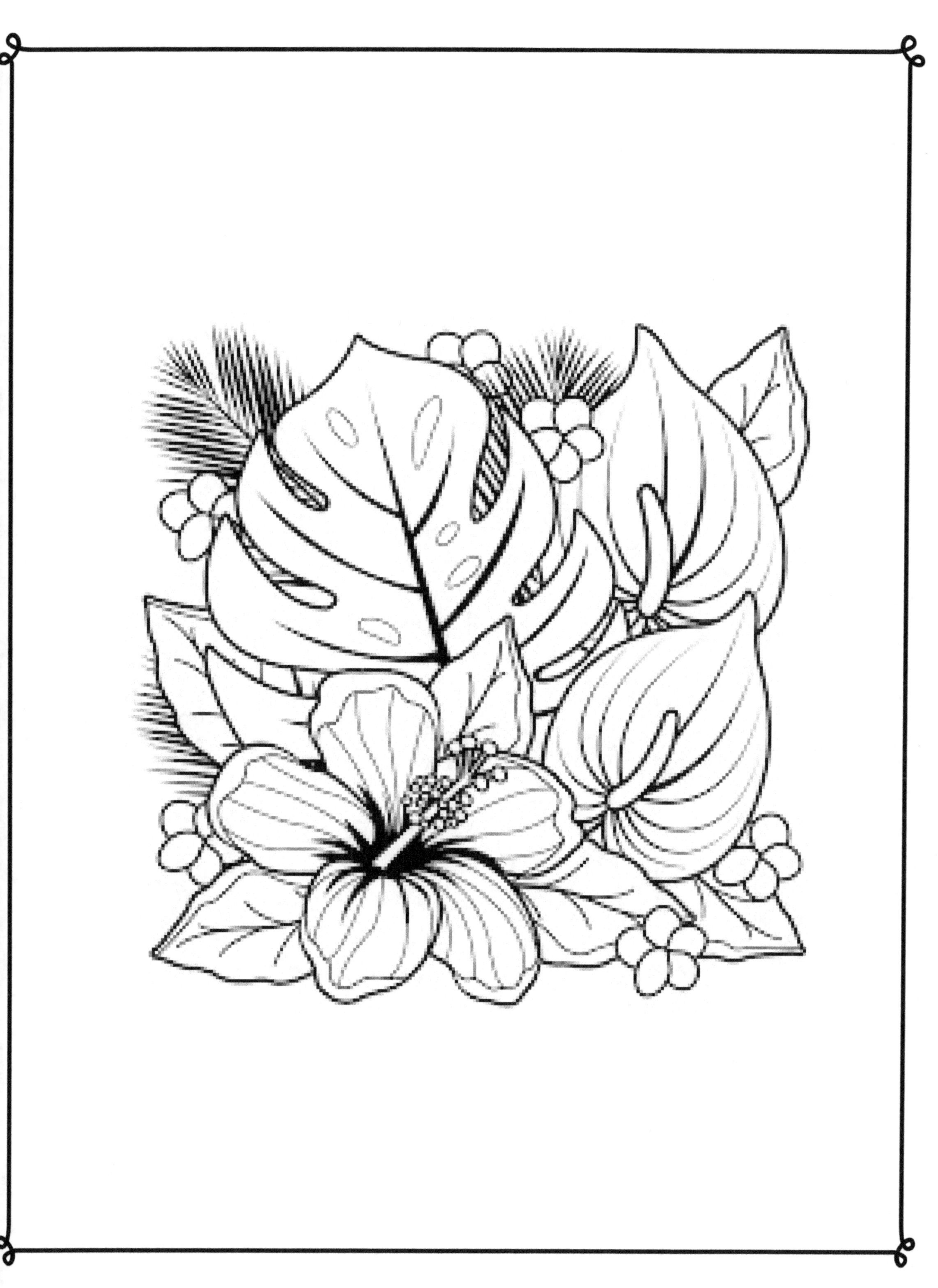

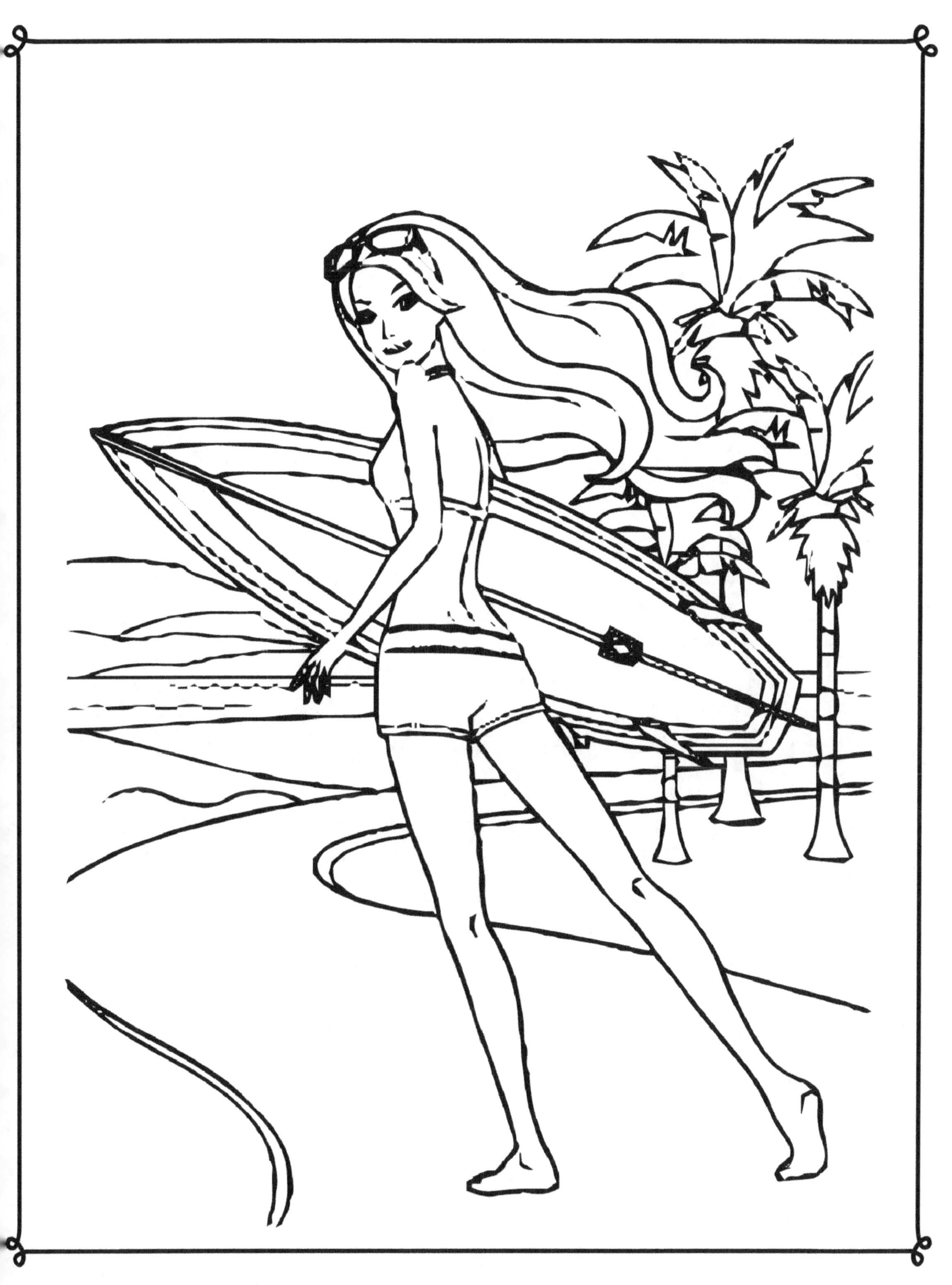

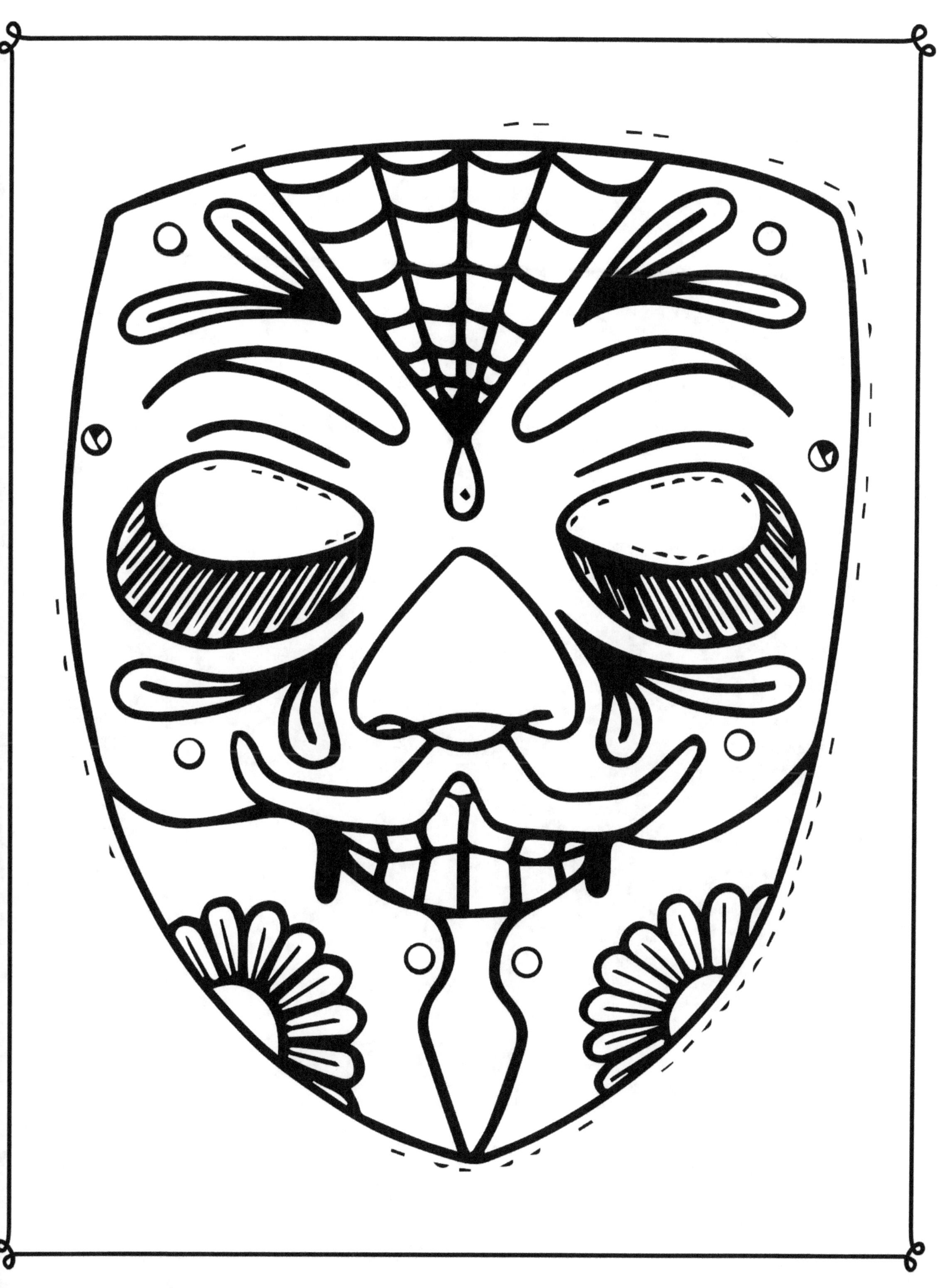

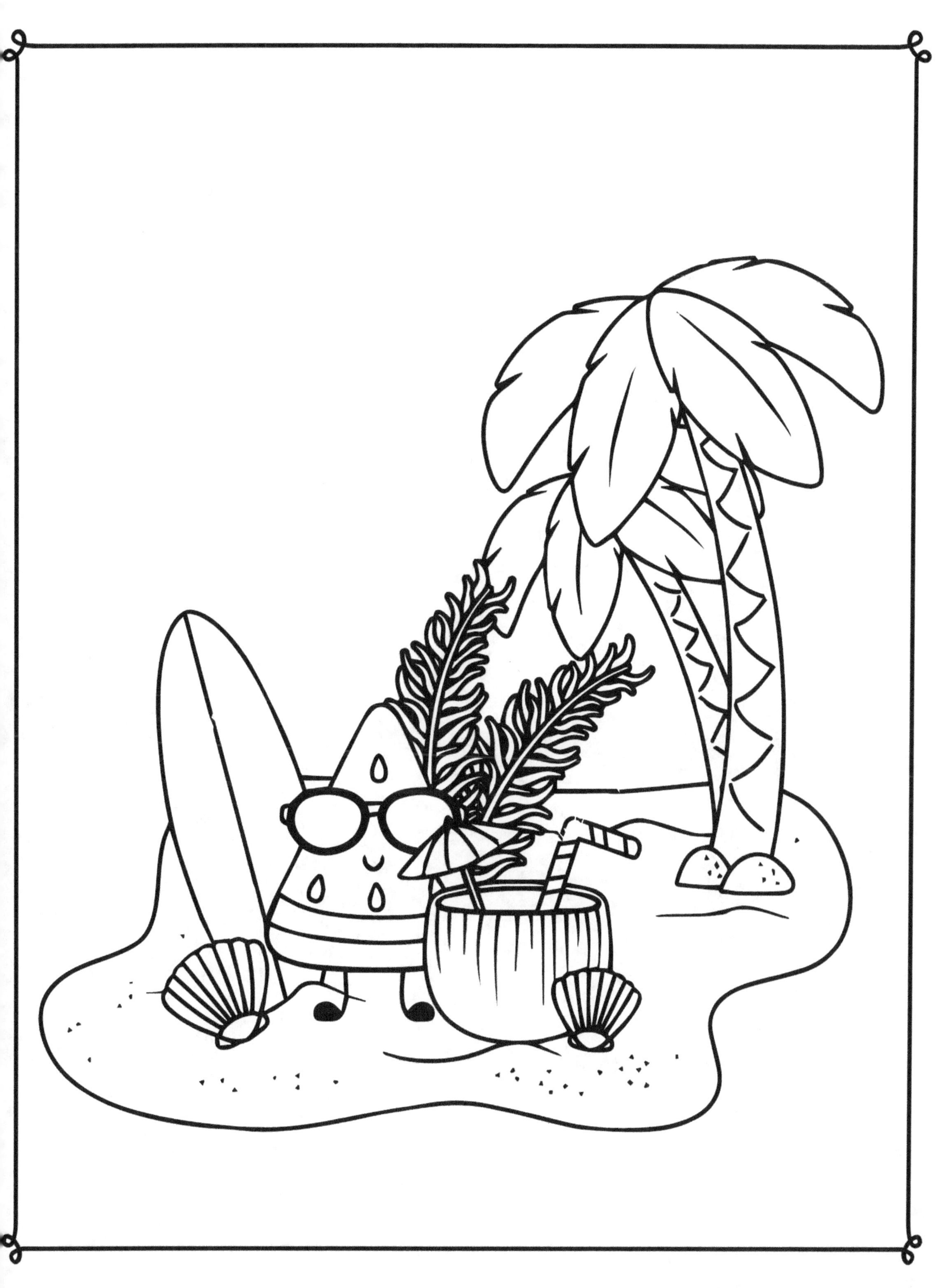

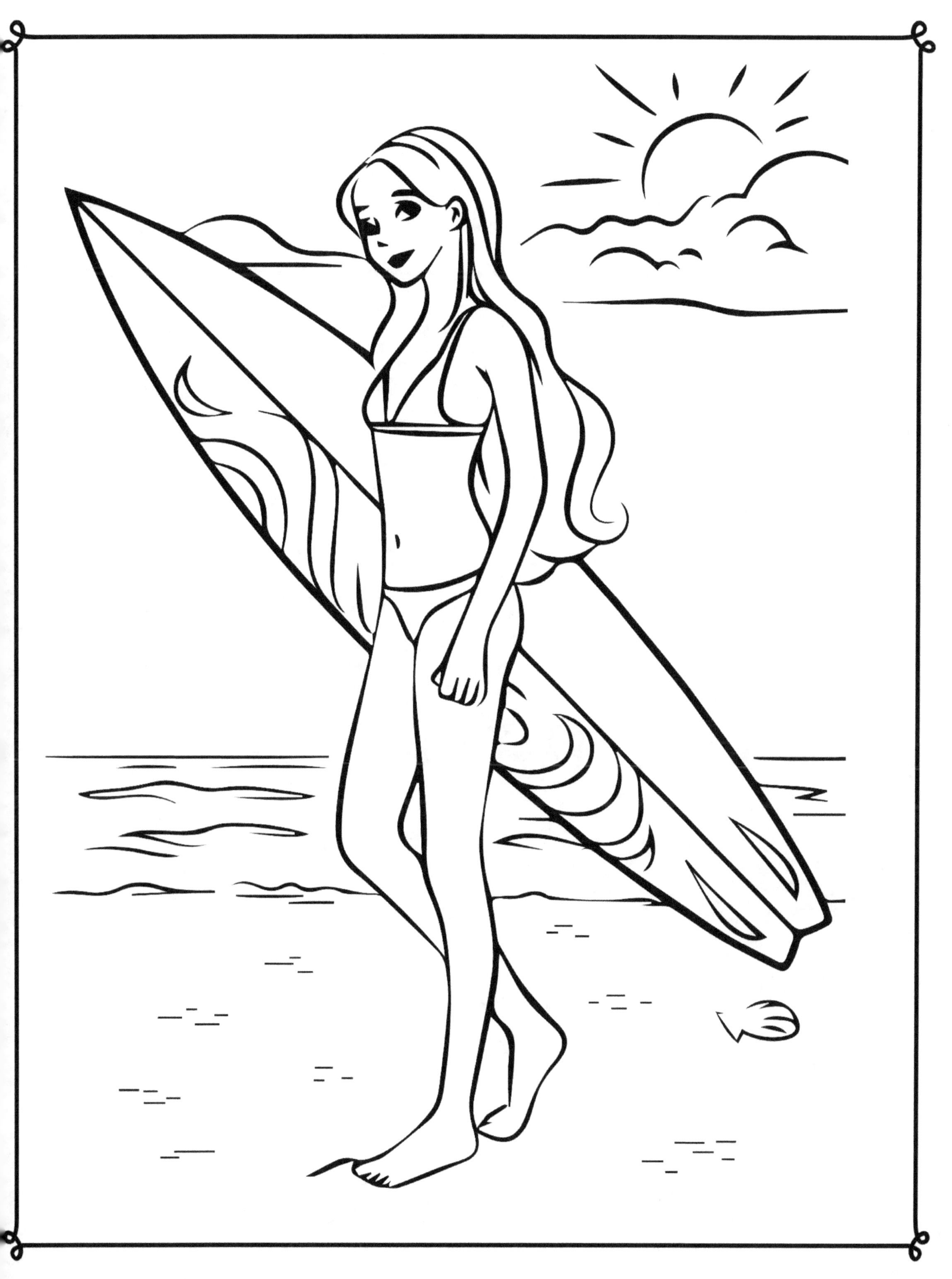

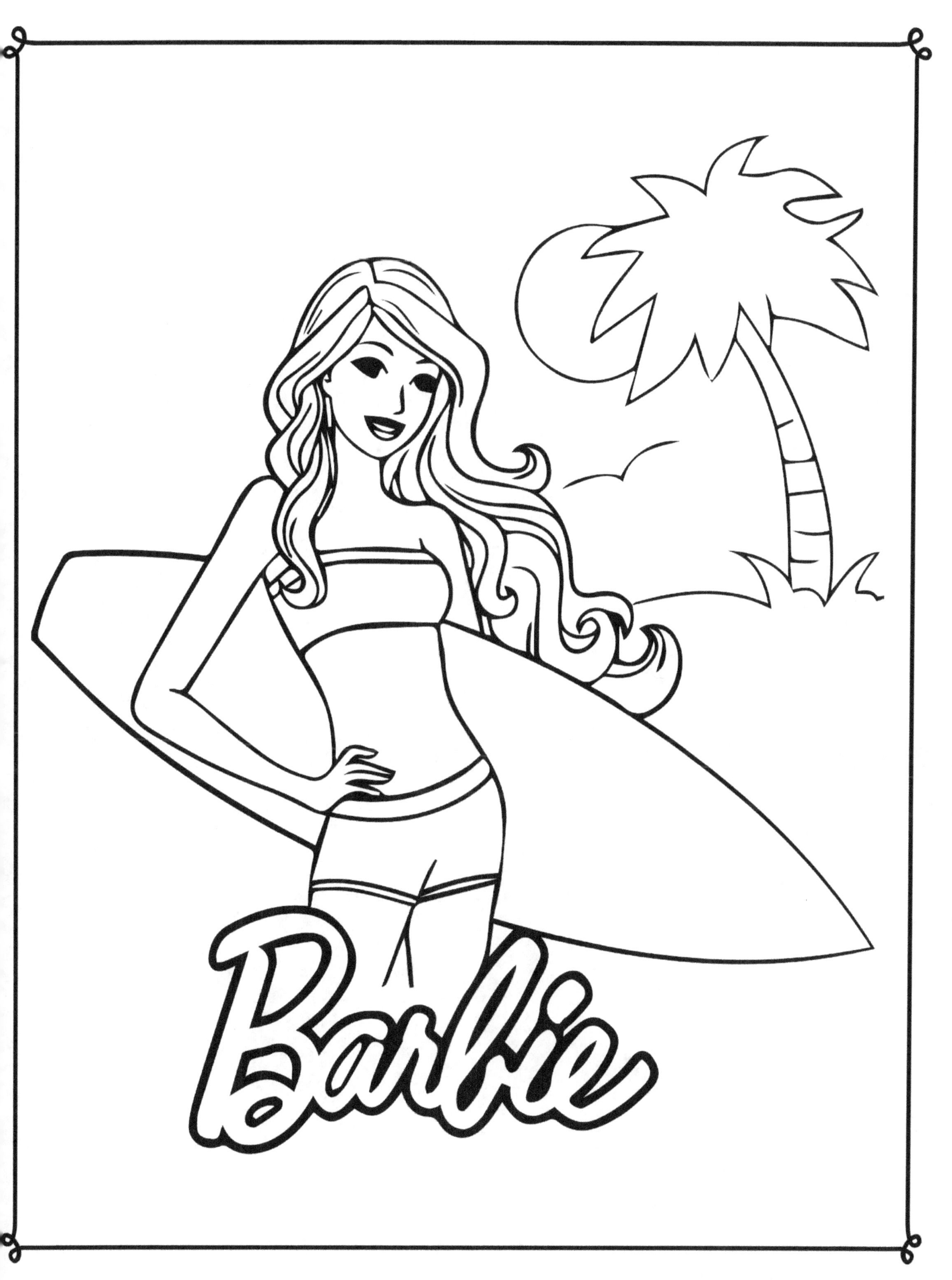

Barbie

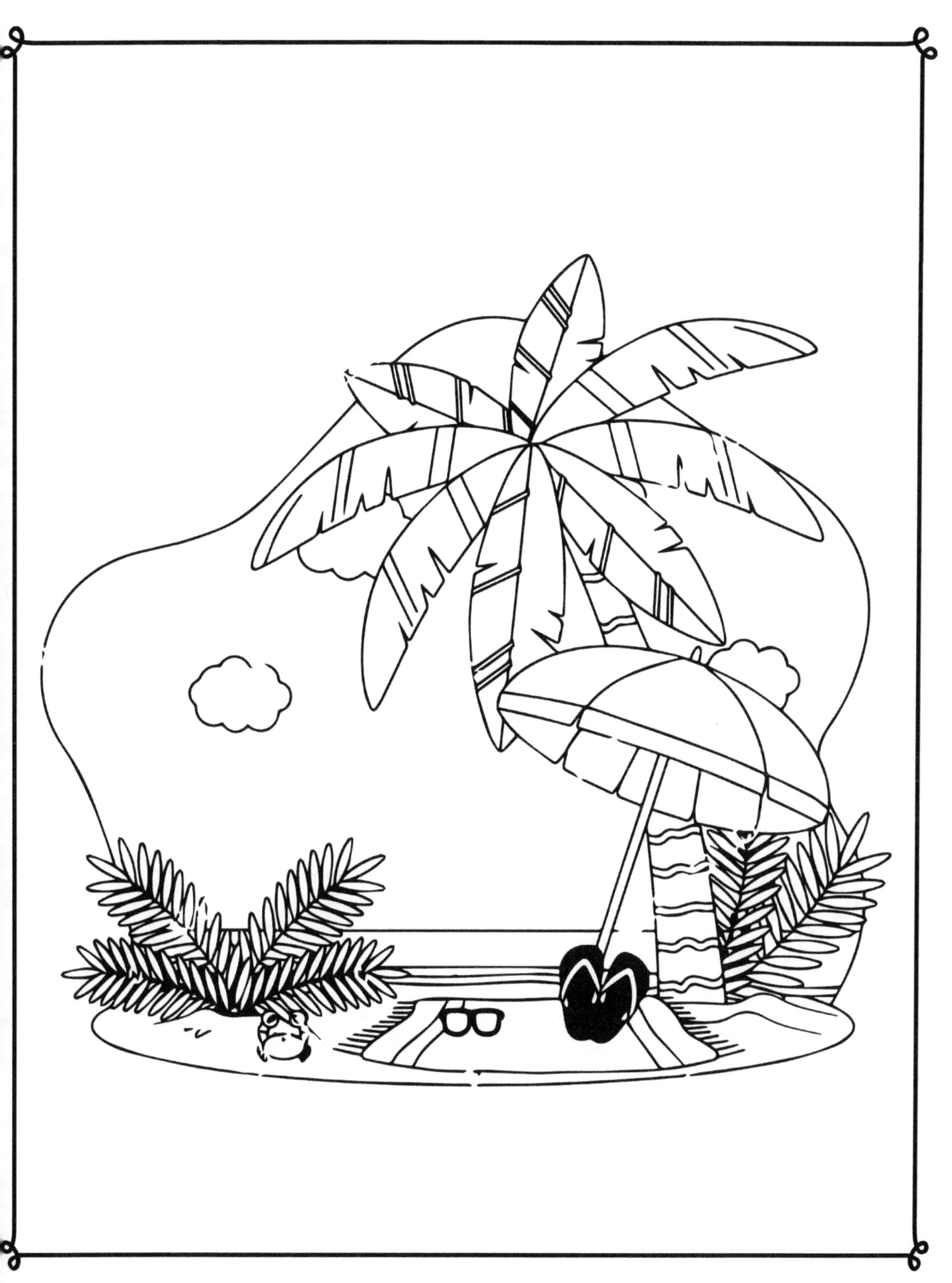

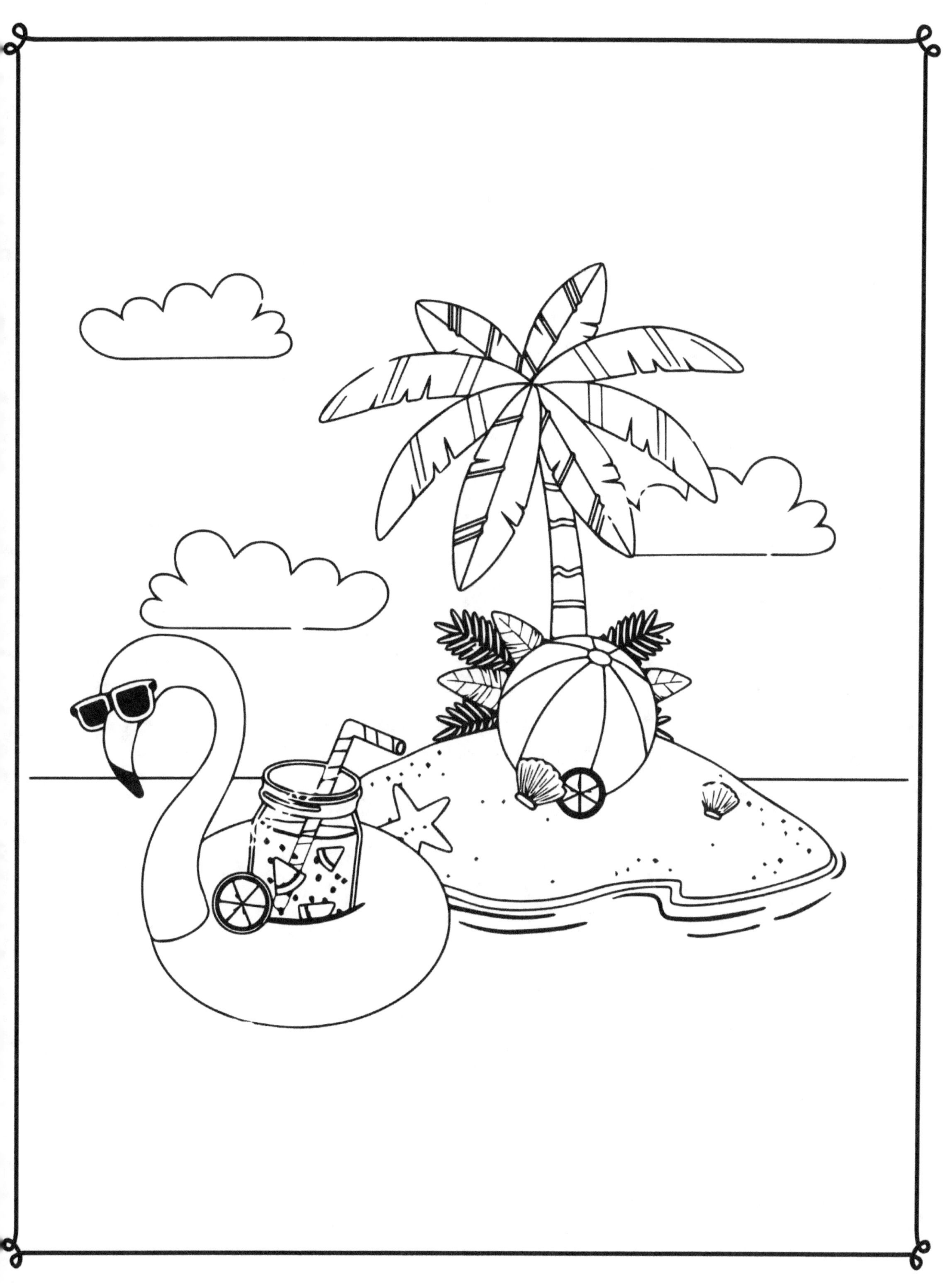

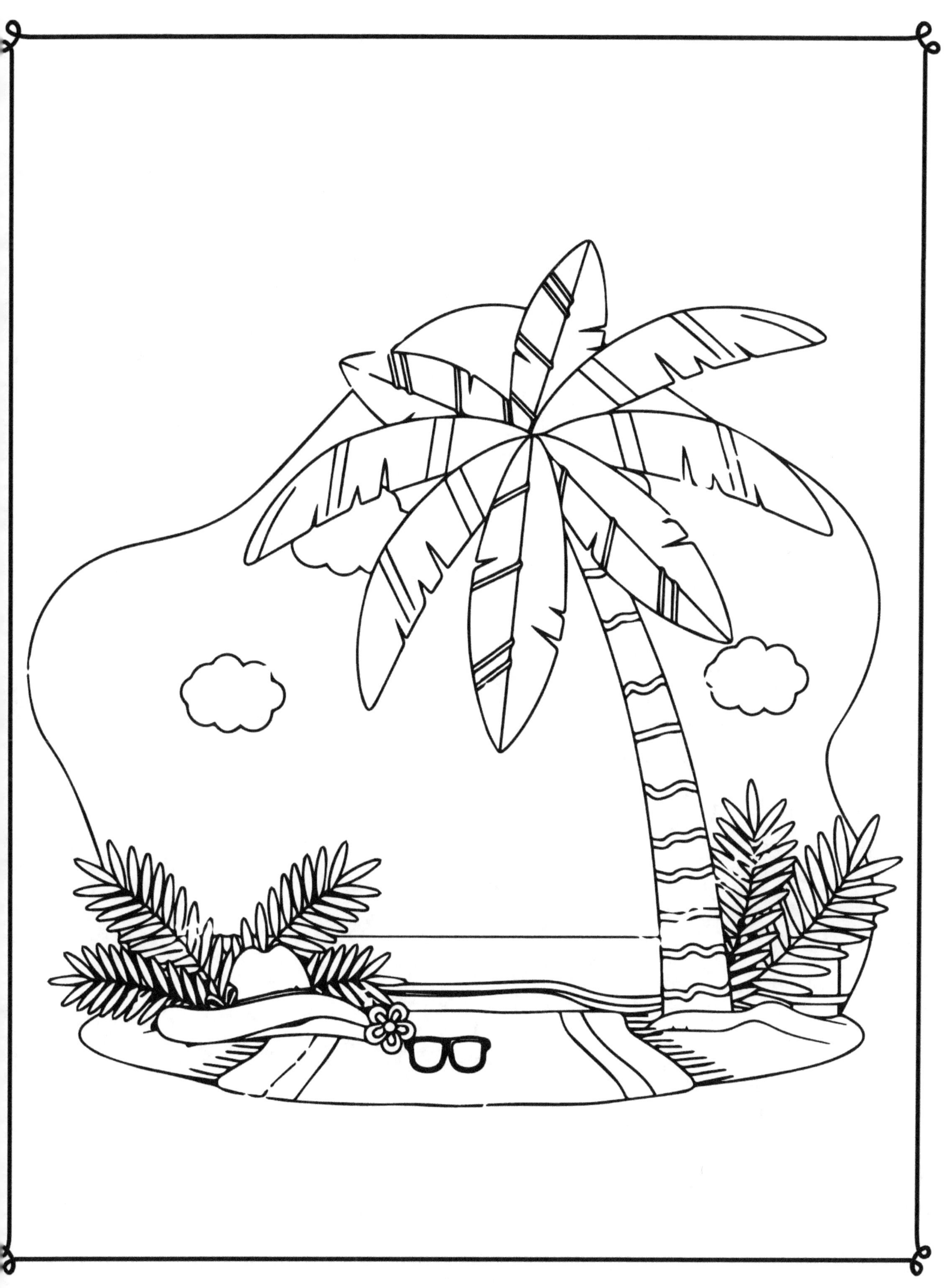

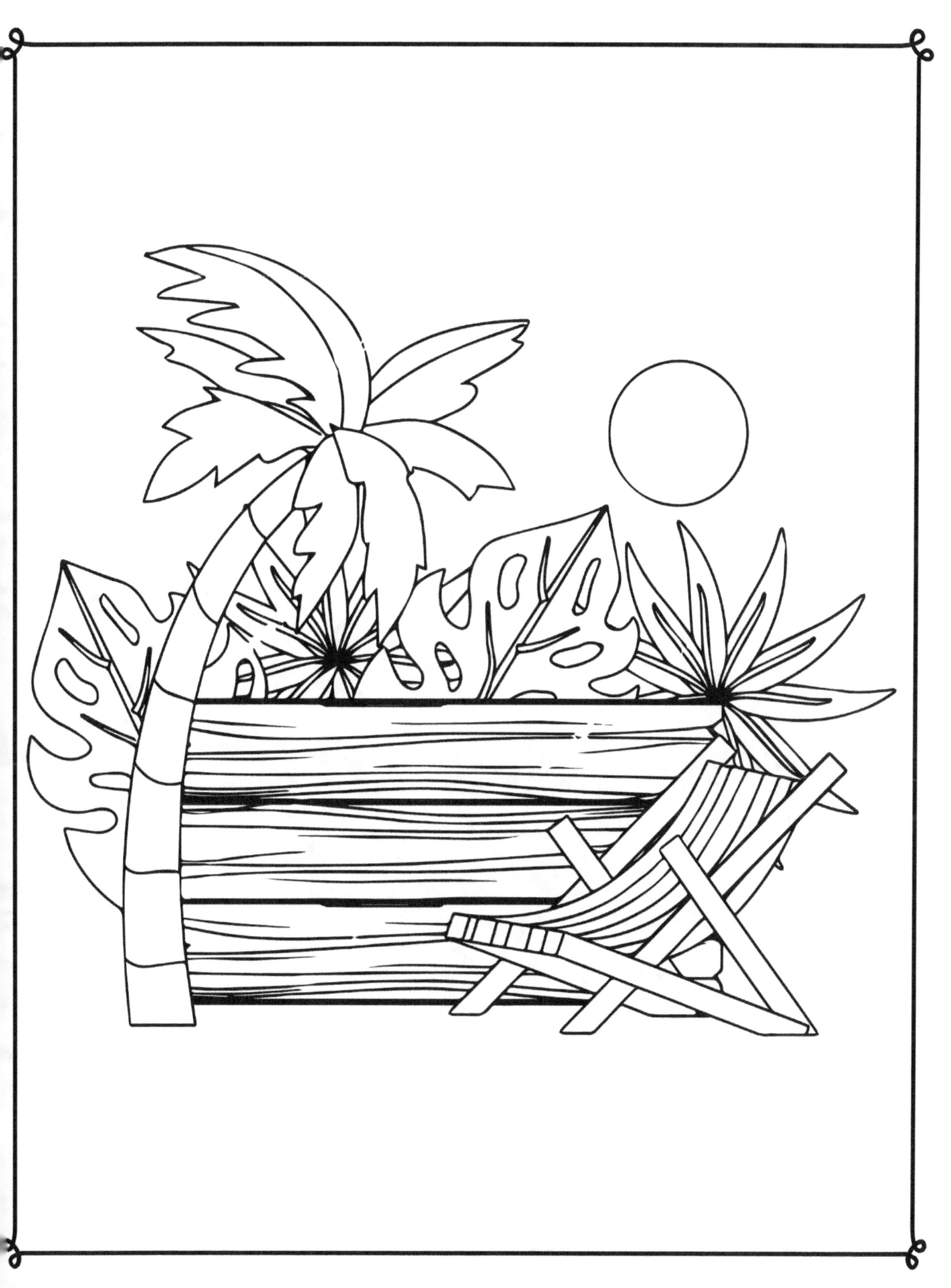

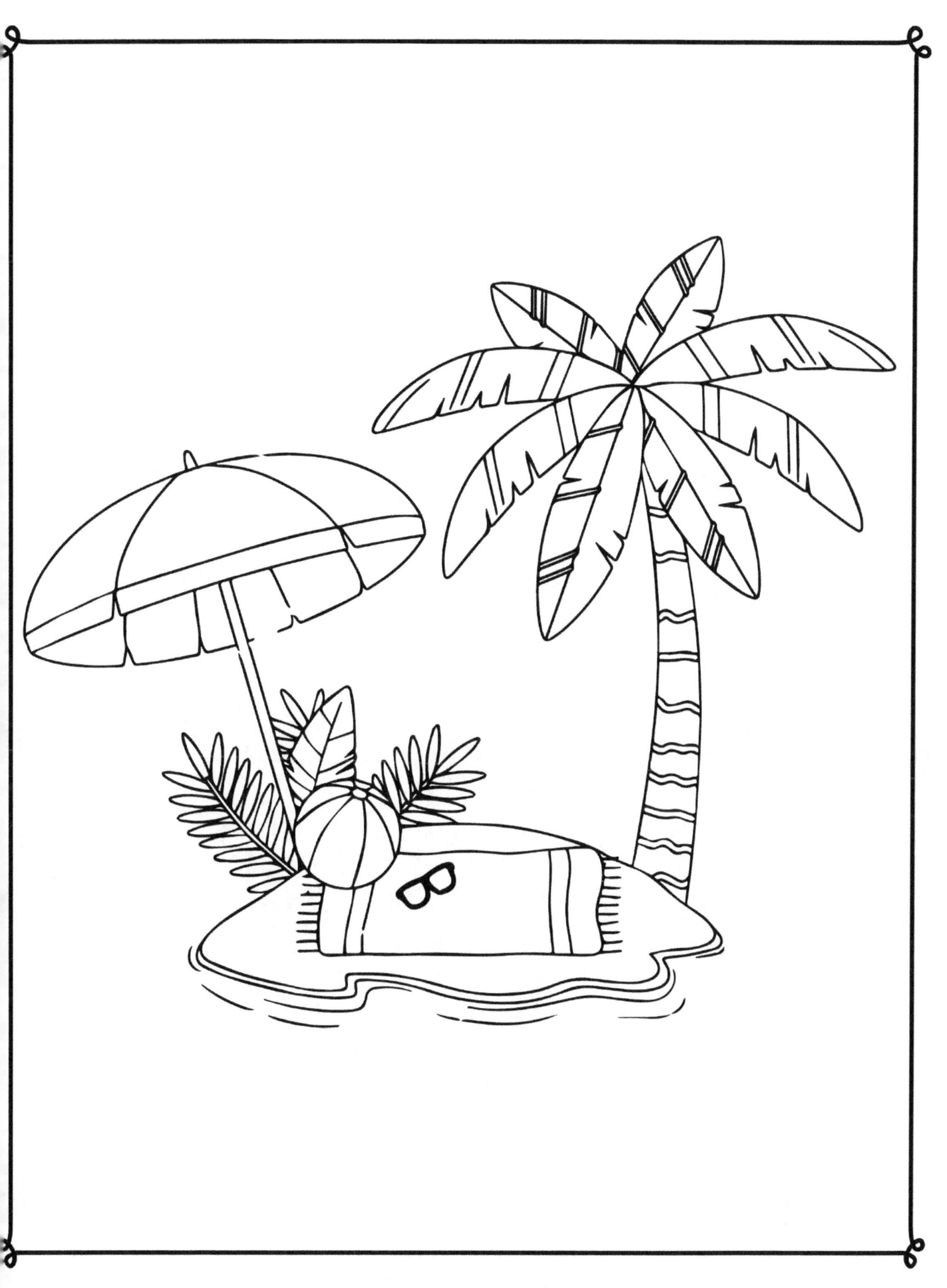

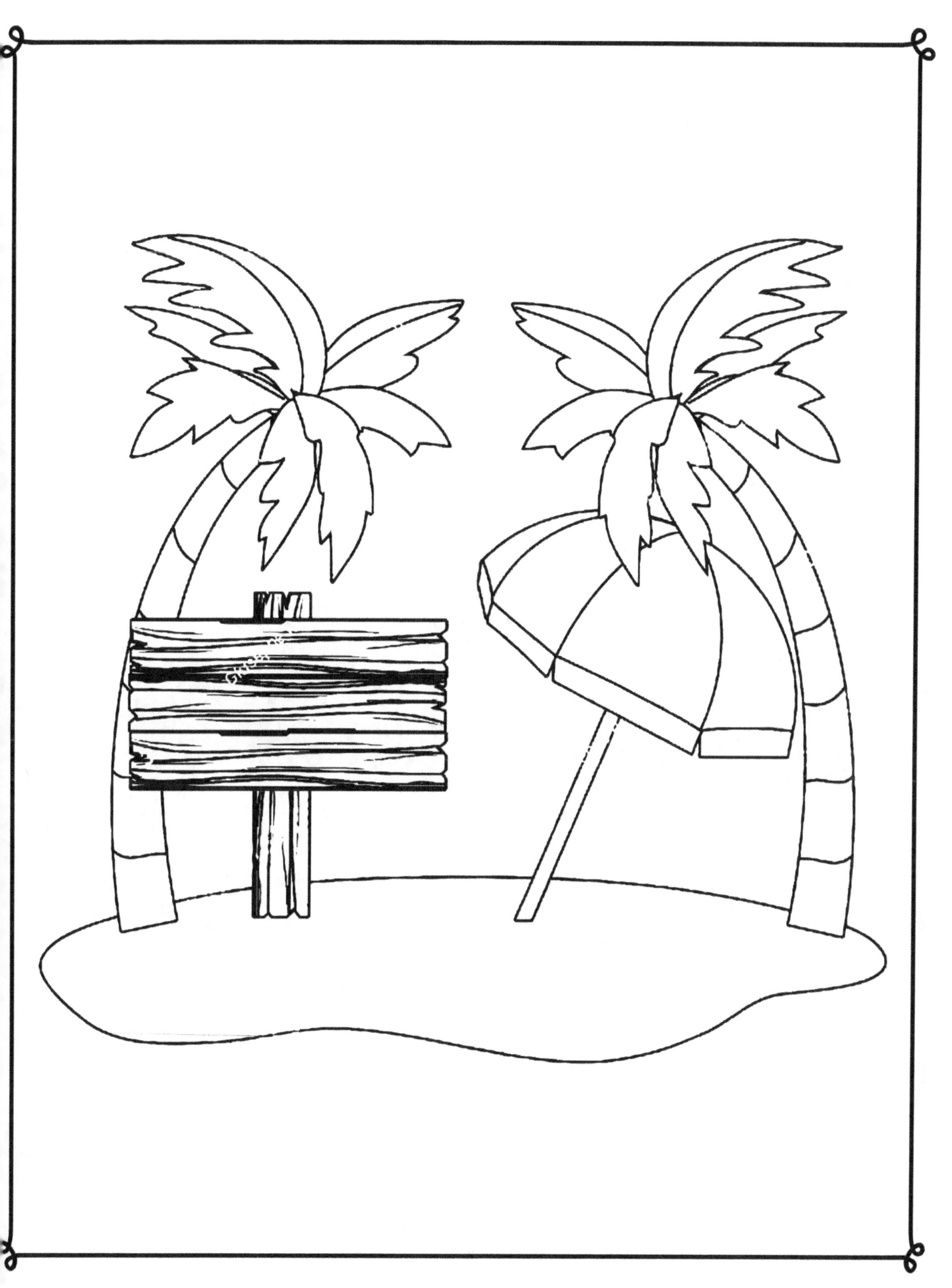

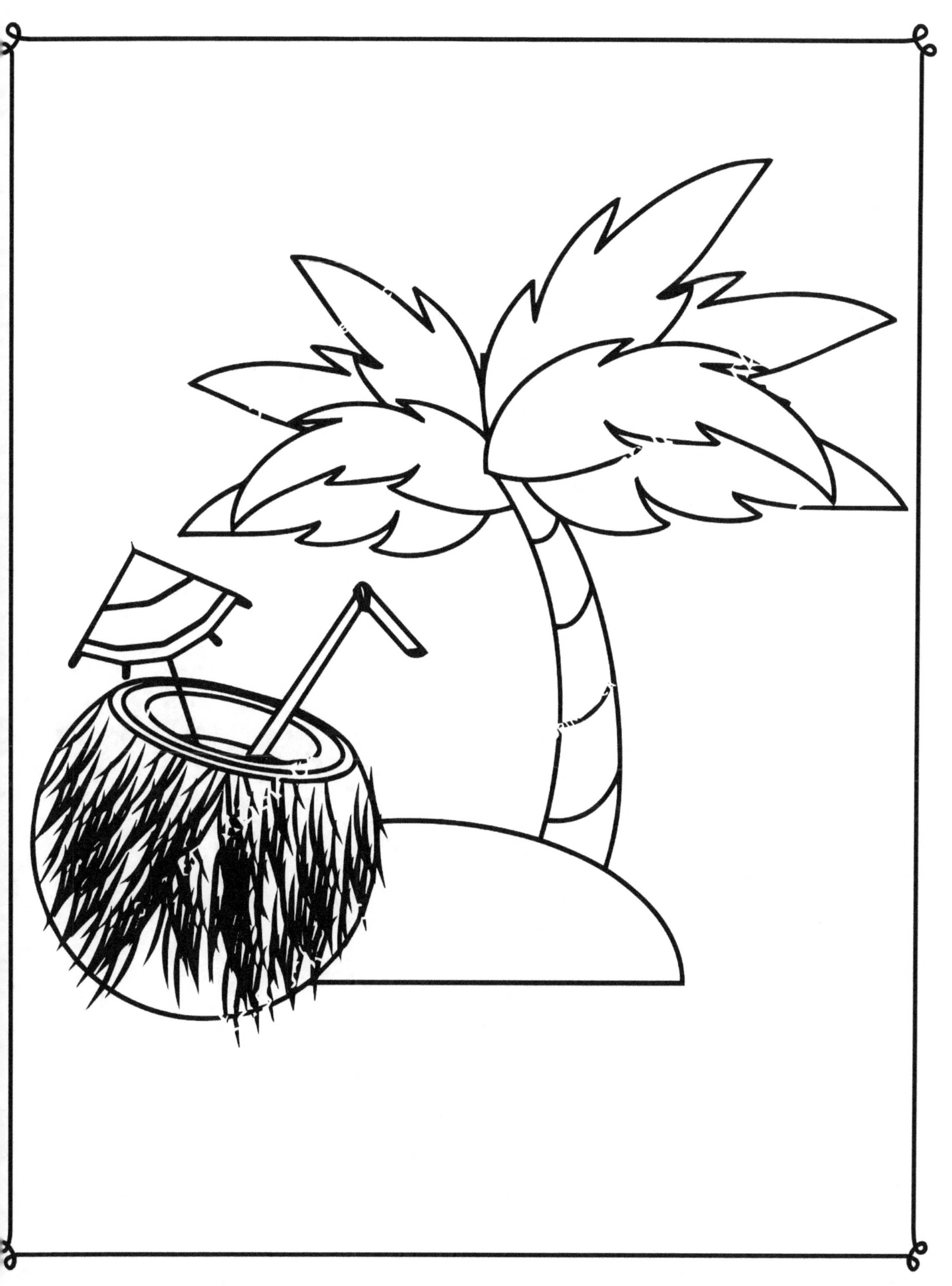

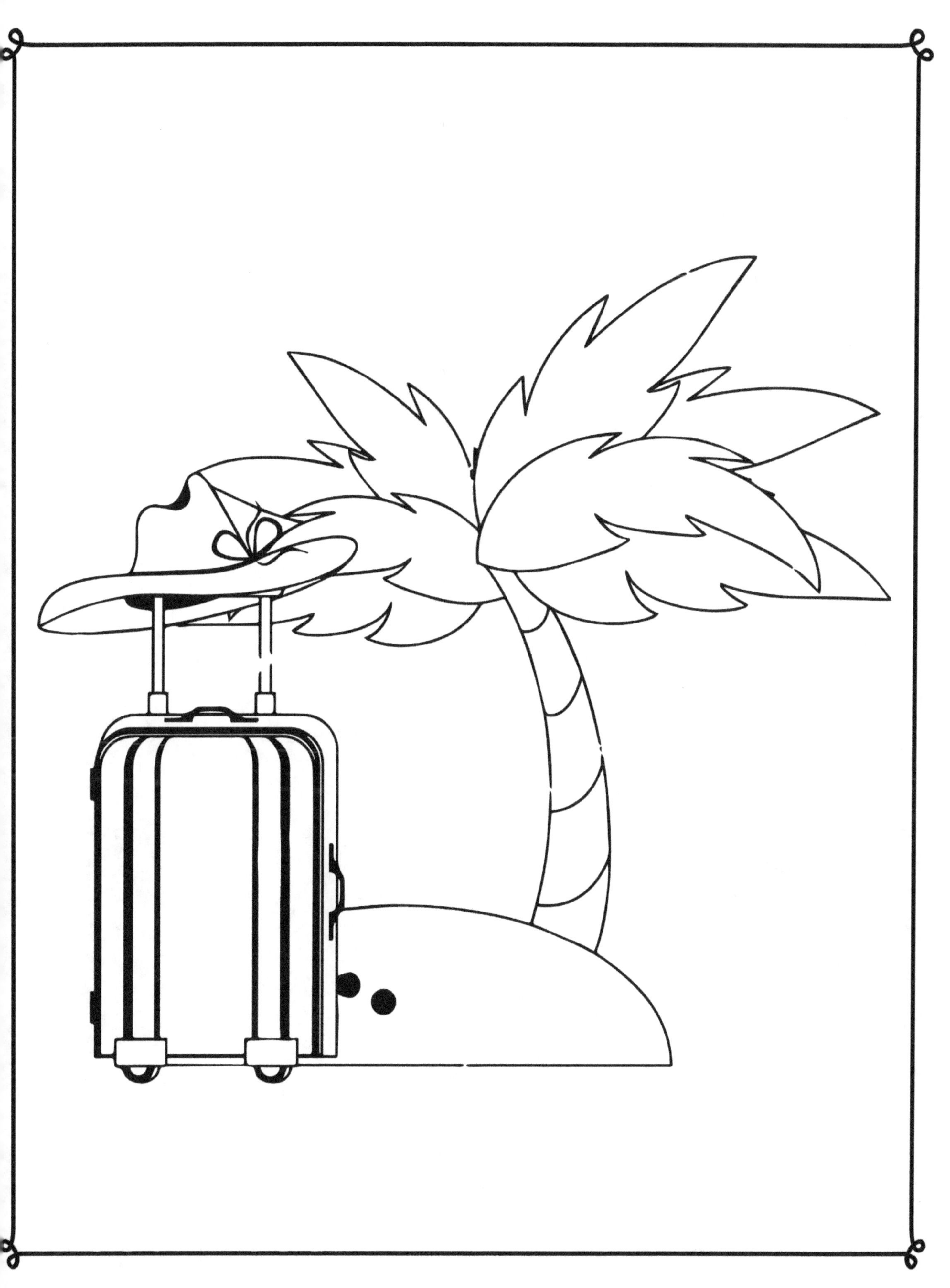

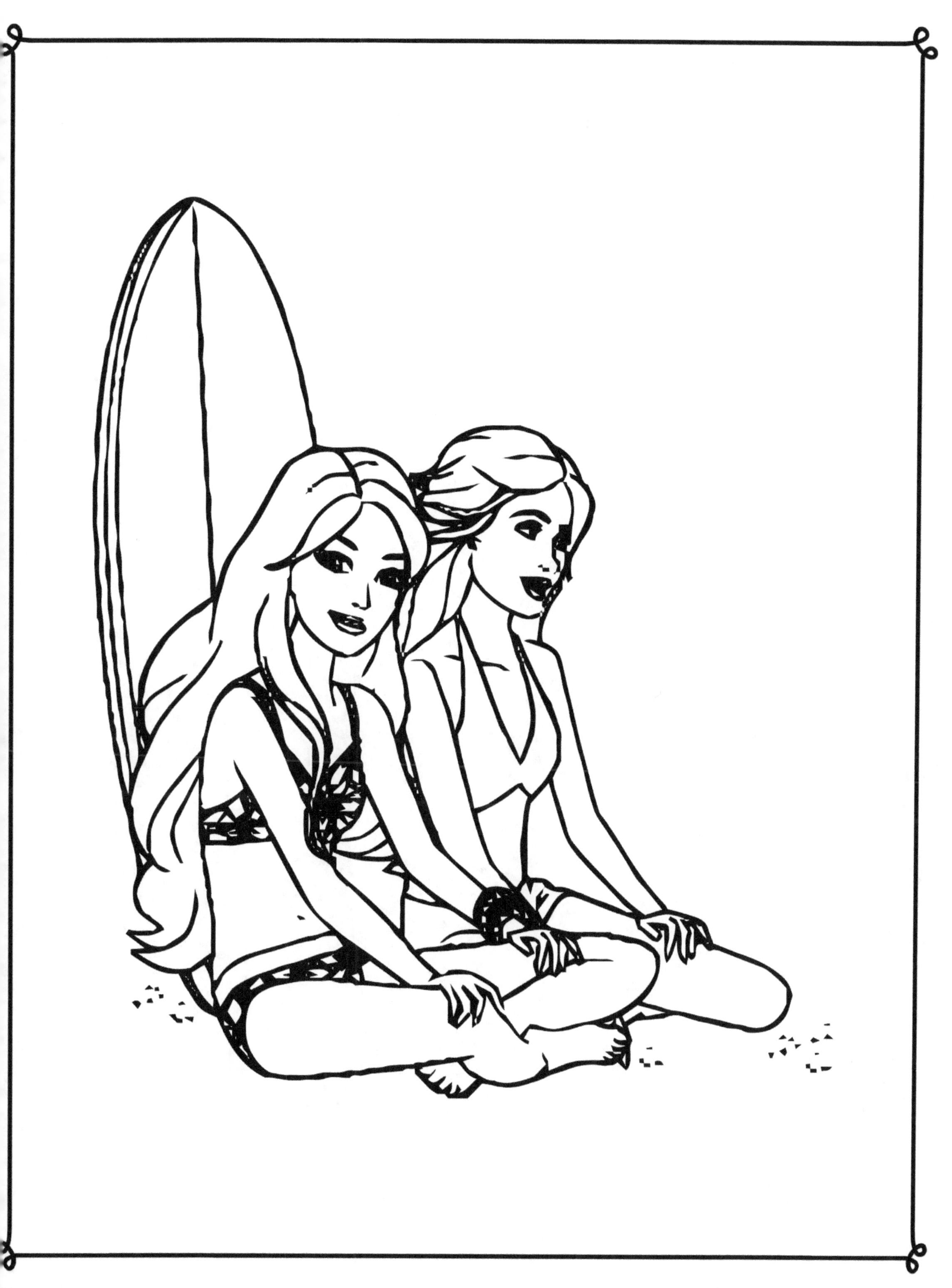

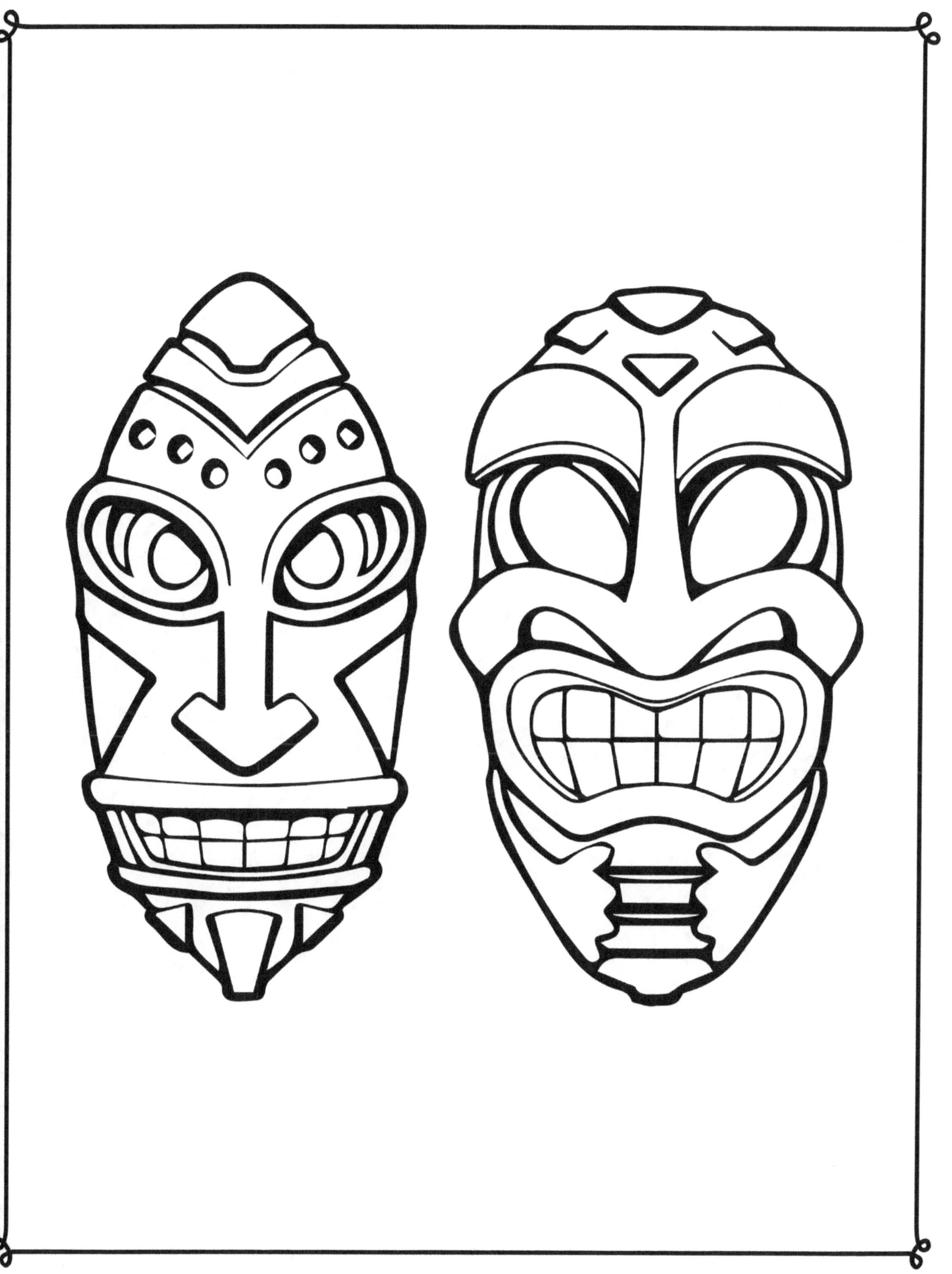

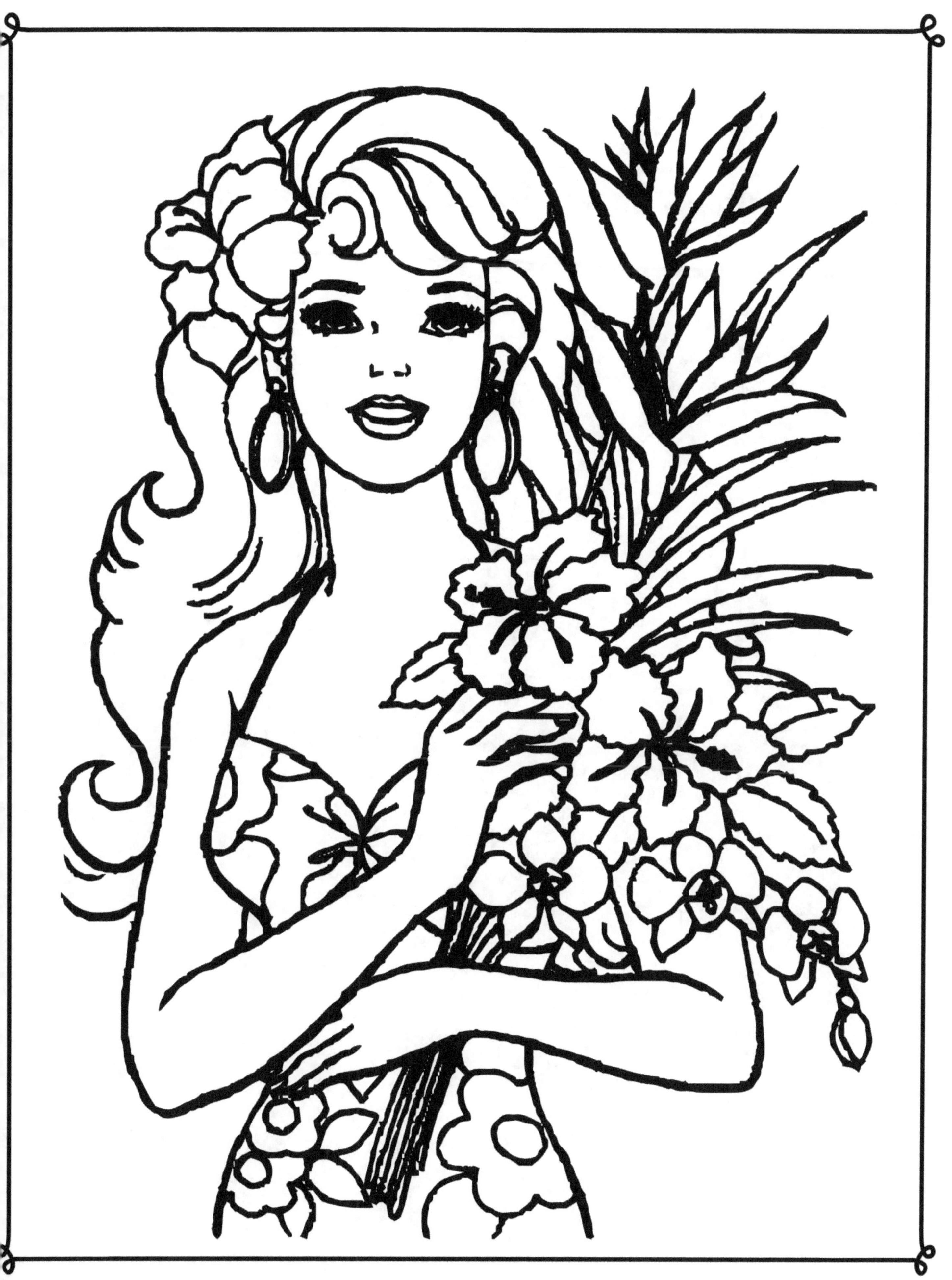

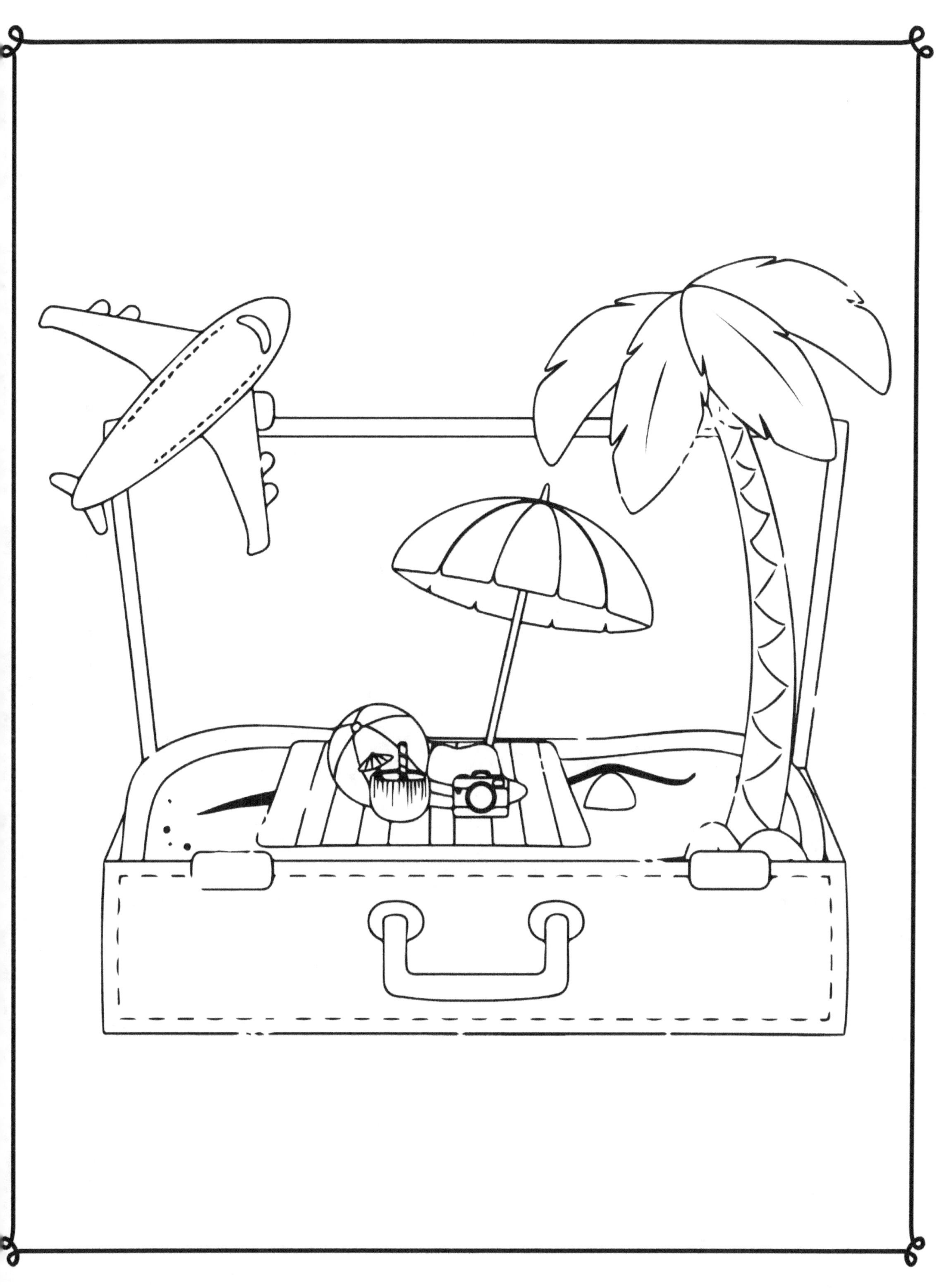

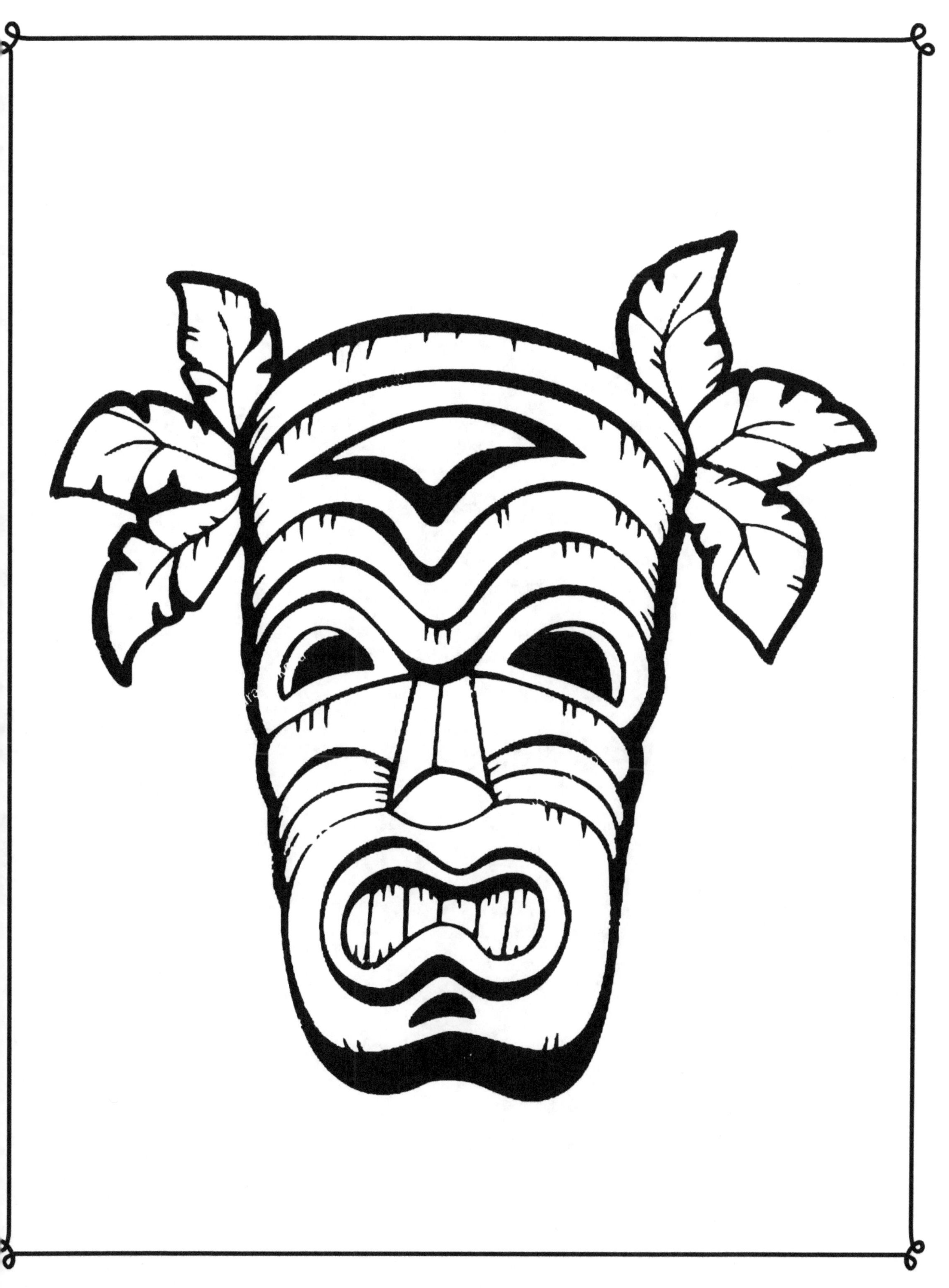

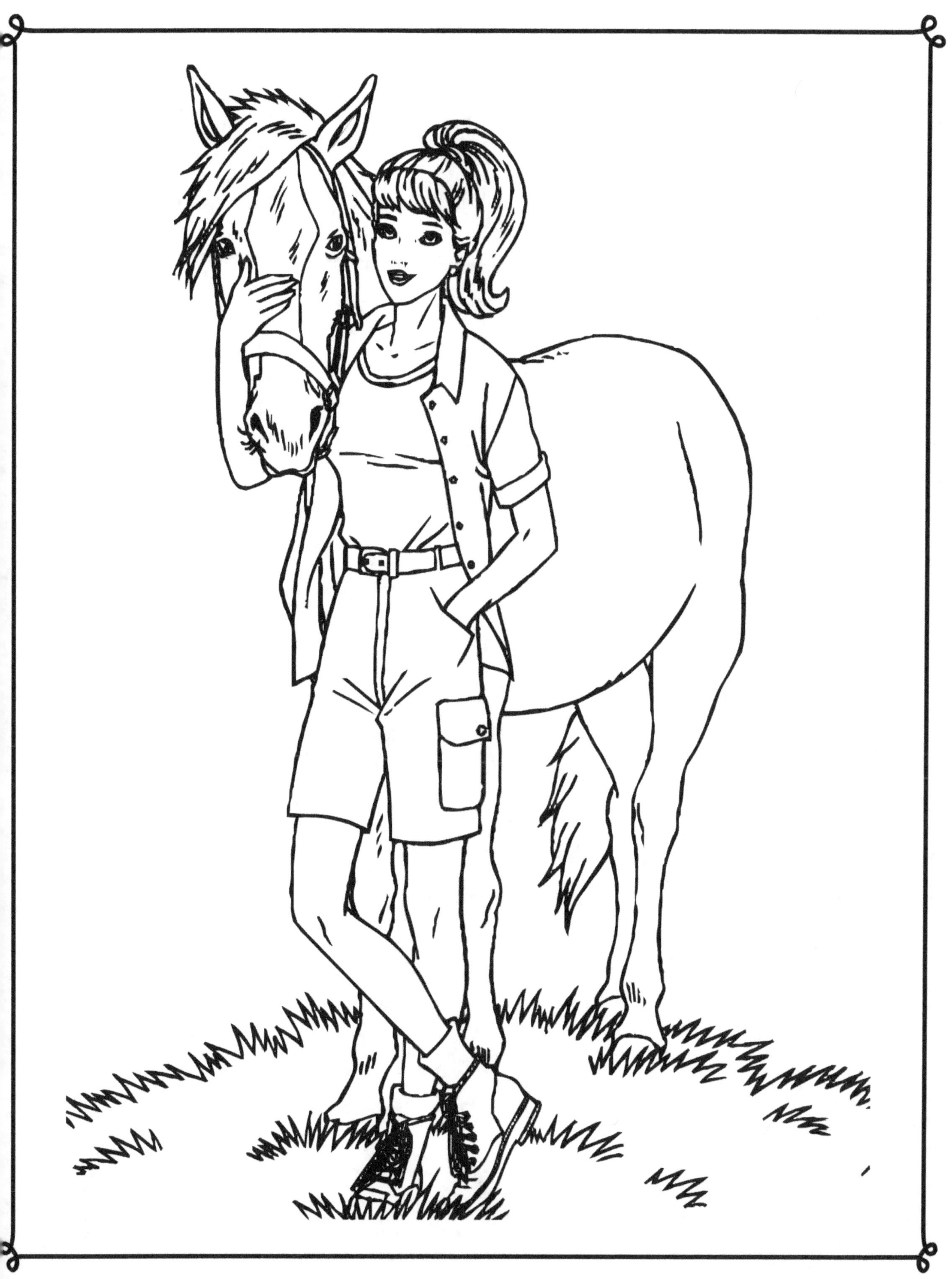

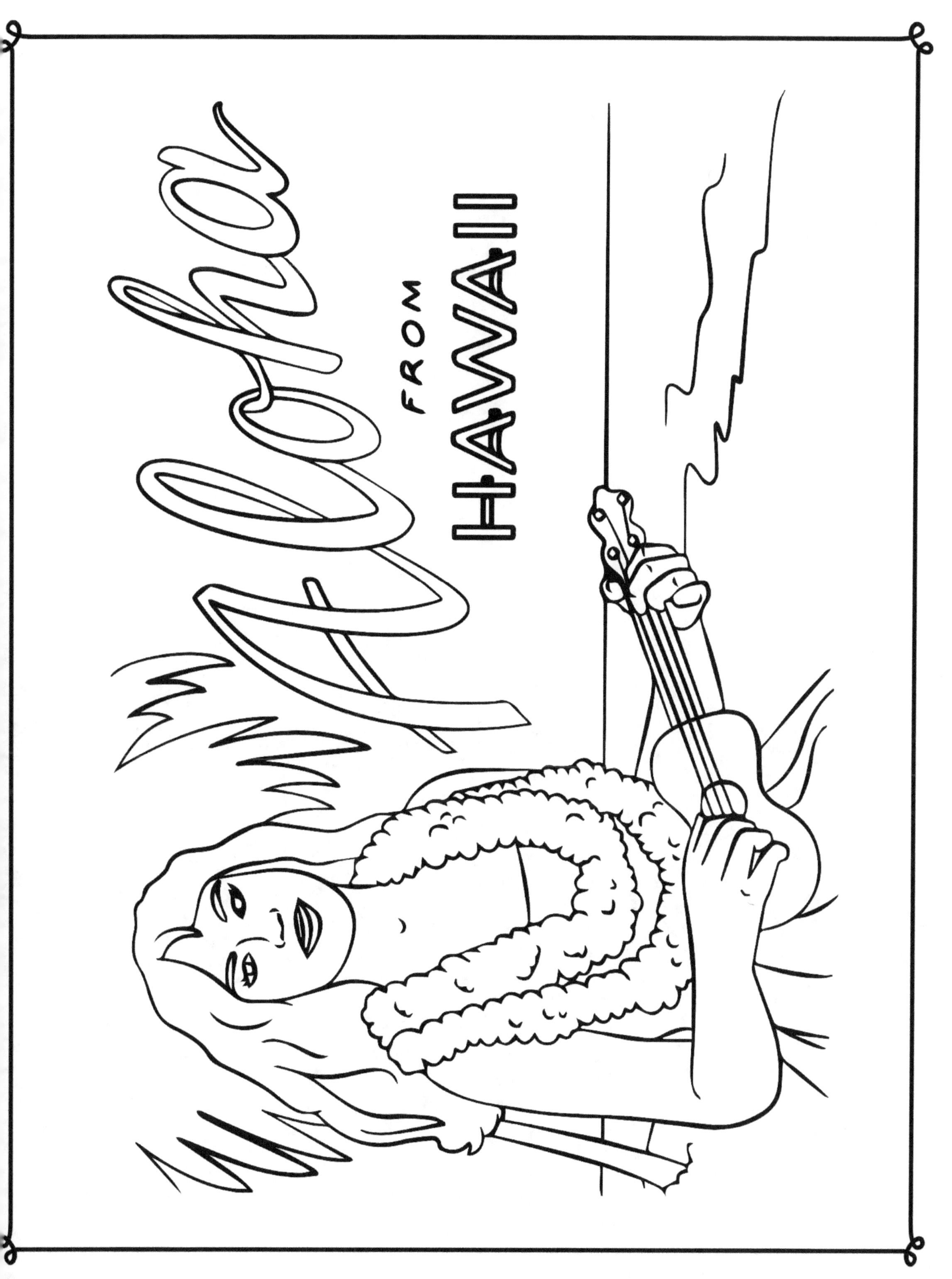

Aloha
FROM HAWAII

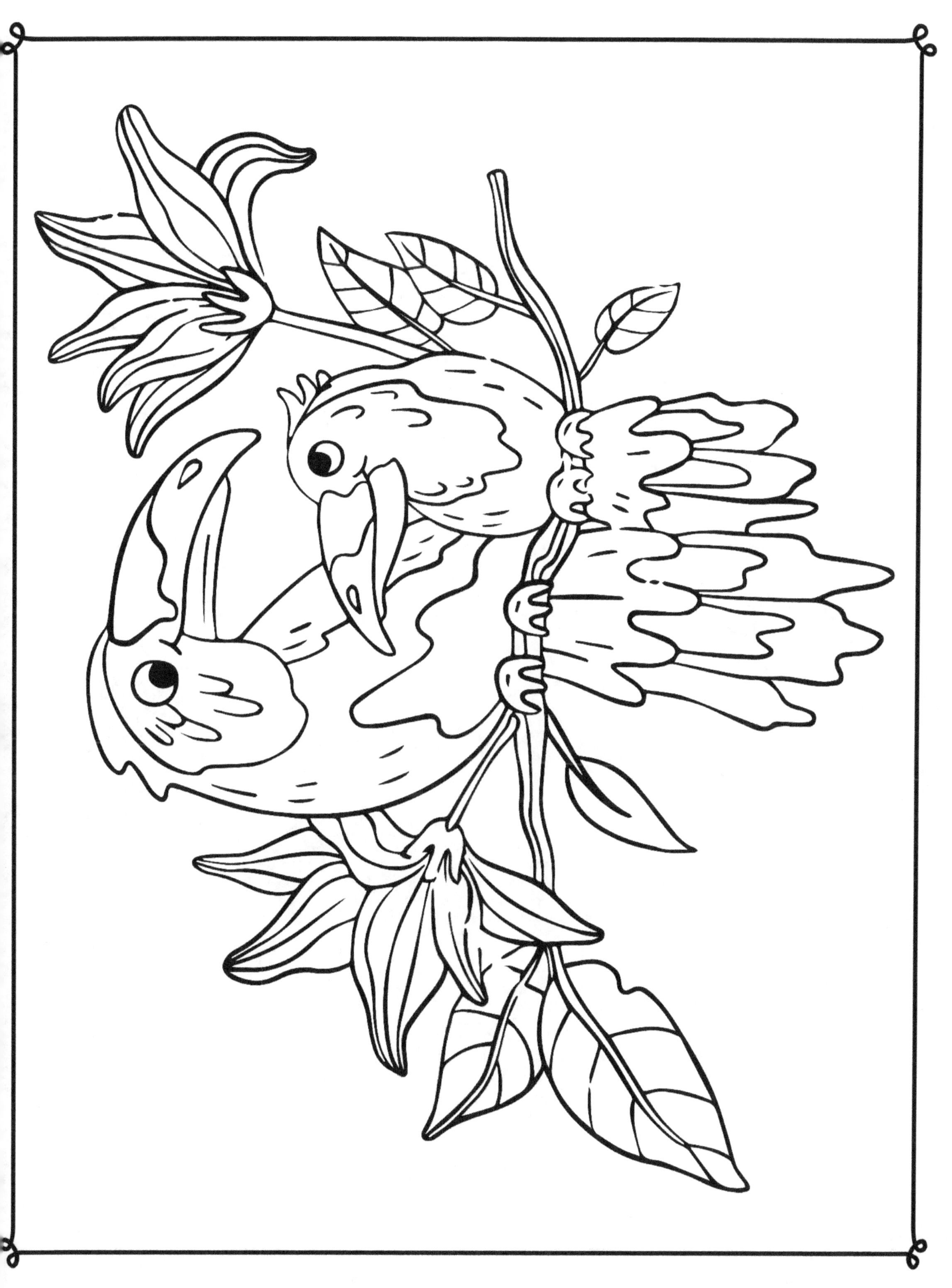

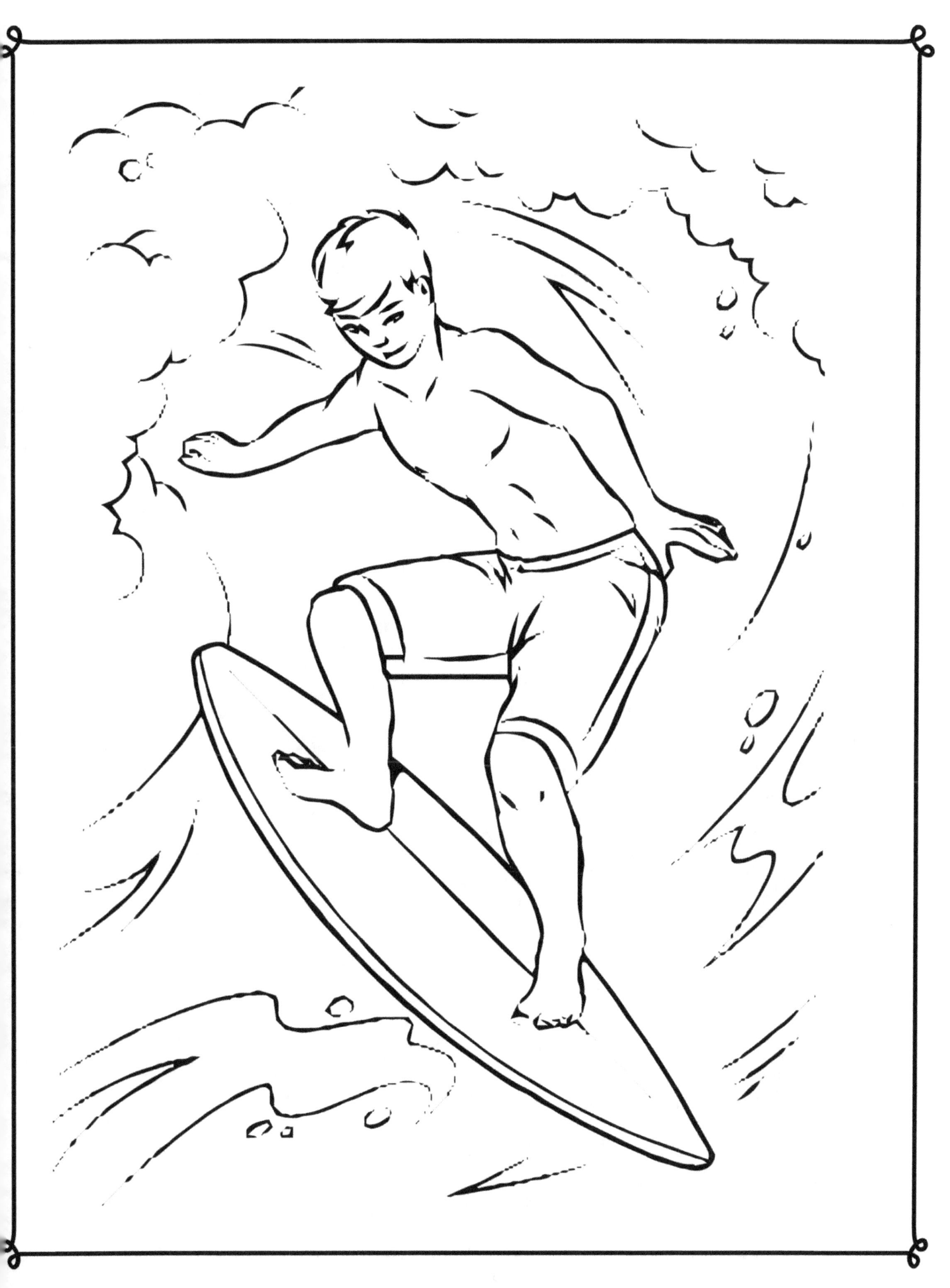

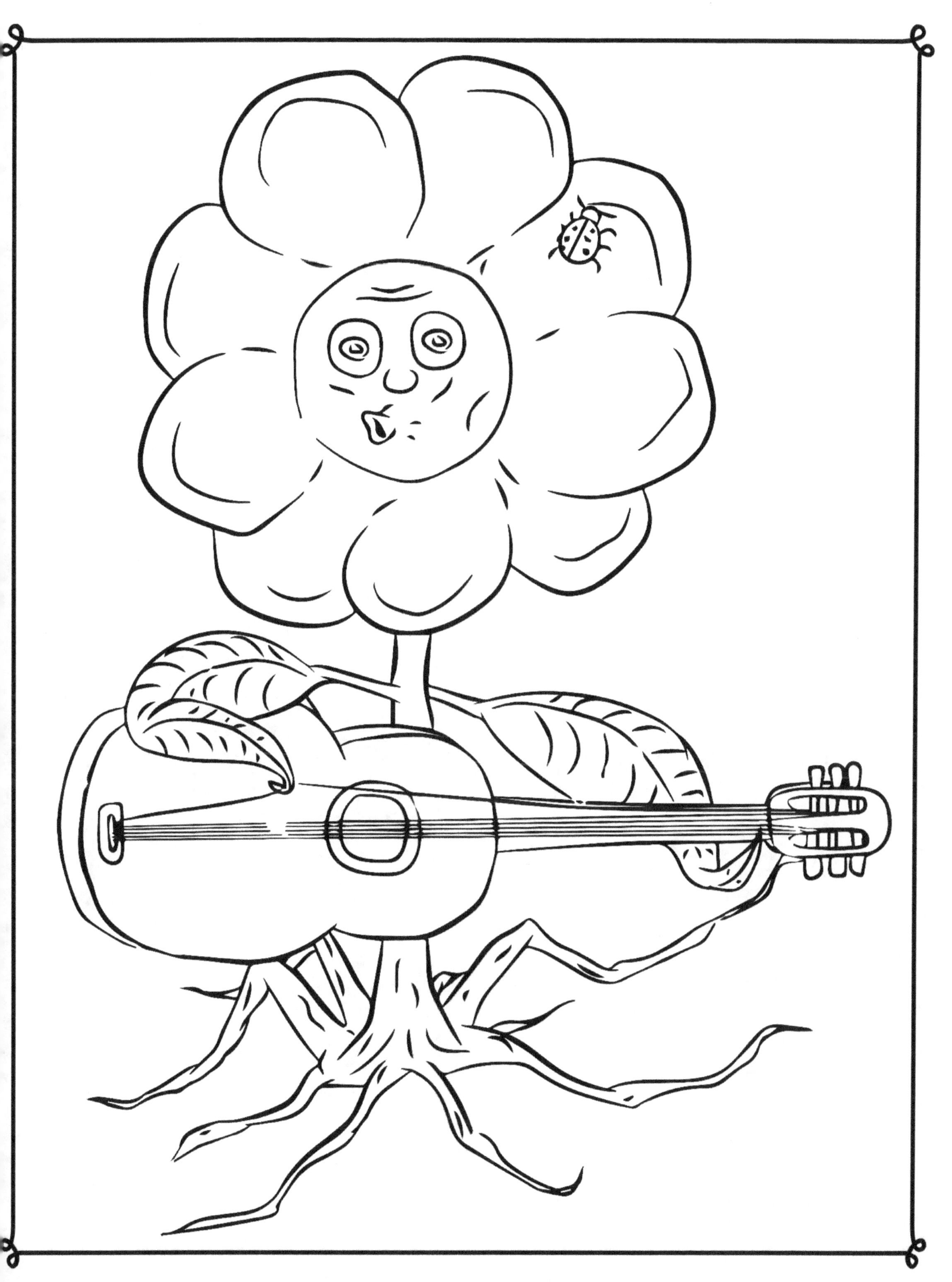

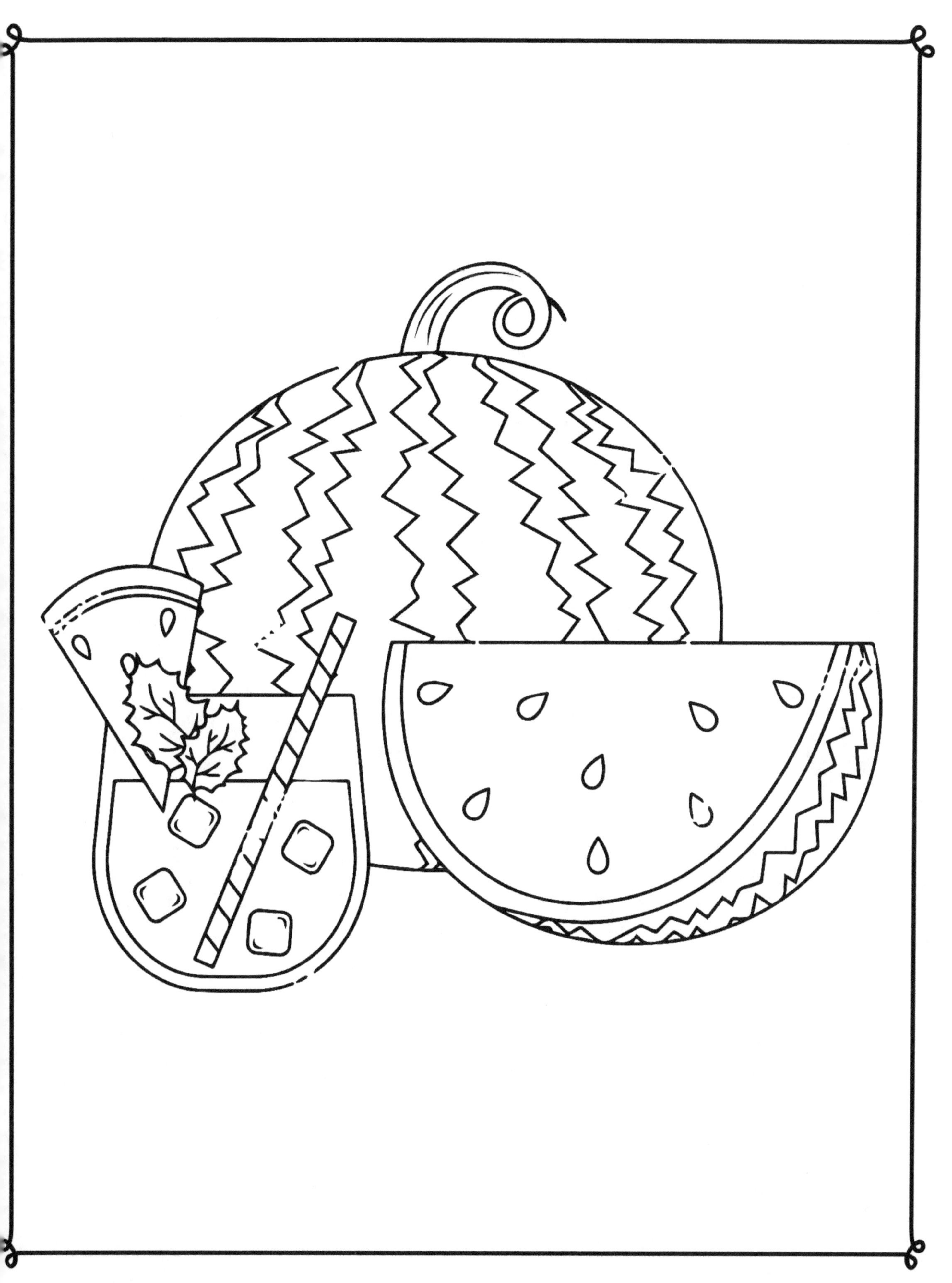

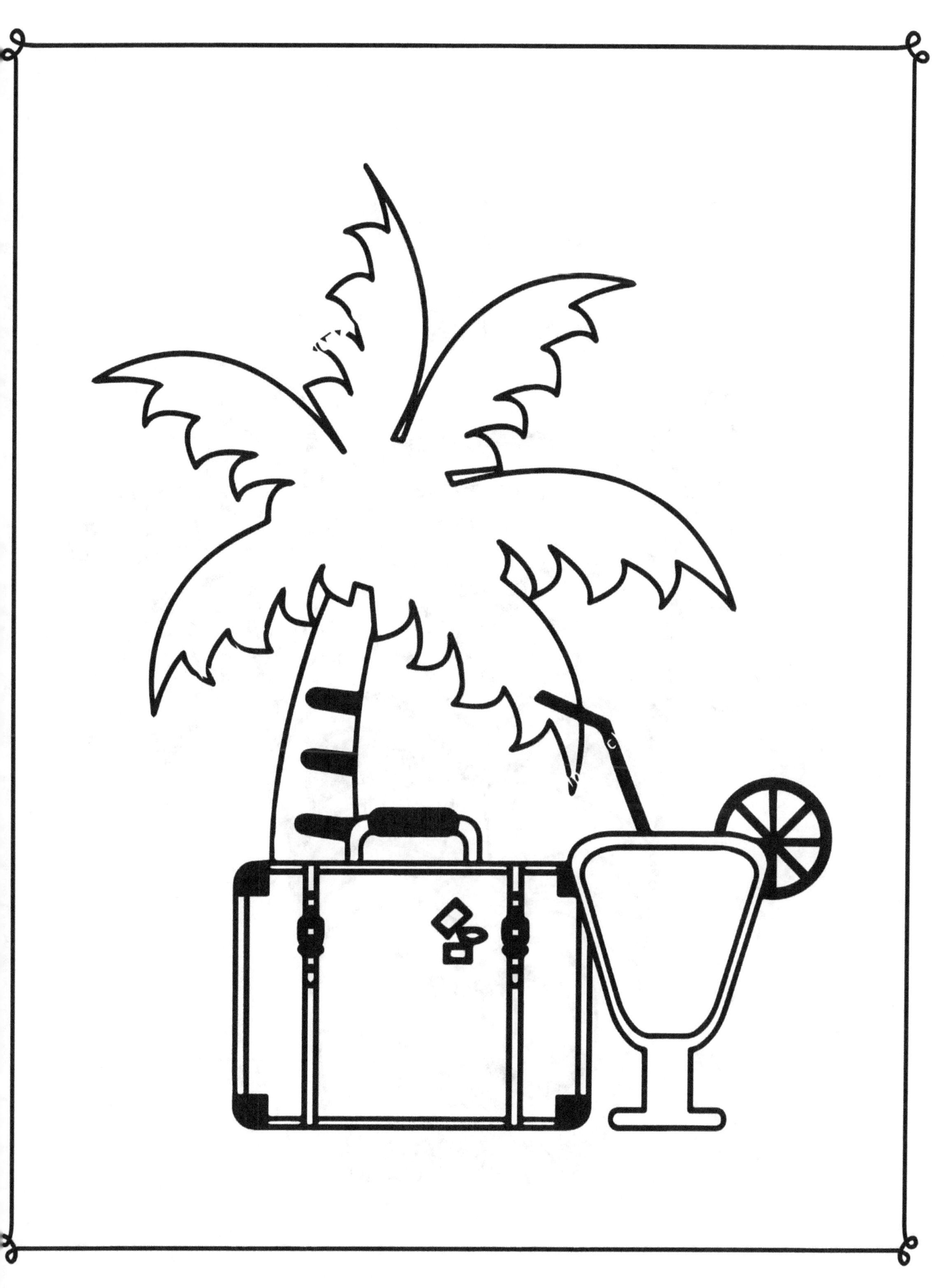

Thanks For Using This Book

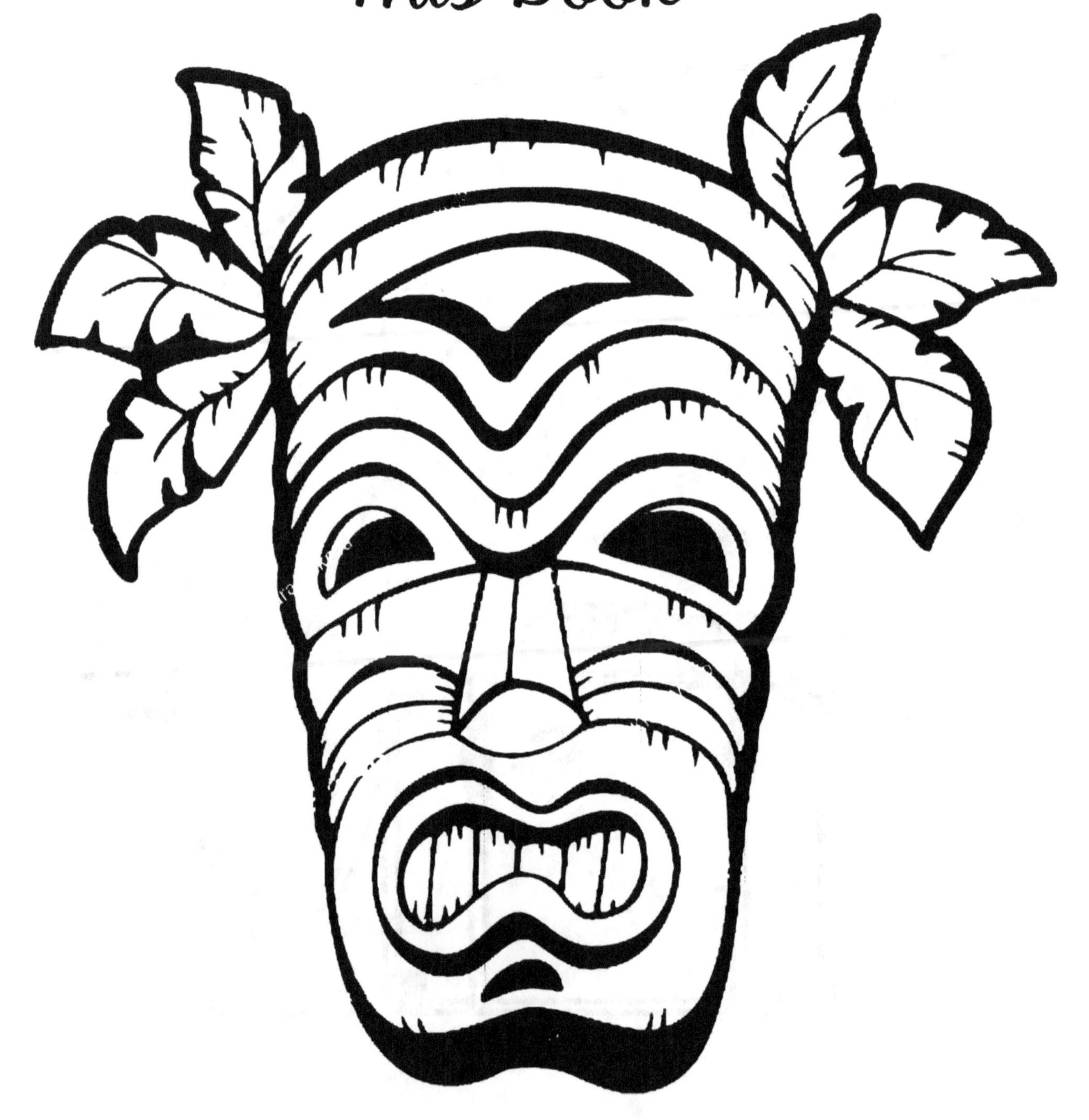

www.ingramcontent.com/pod-product-compliance
Lightning Source LLC
Chambersburg PA
CBHW081722250726
48657CB00010B/3090